MW01641353

ADVANCED MEDICAL SYSTEMS:

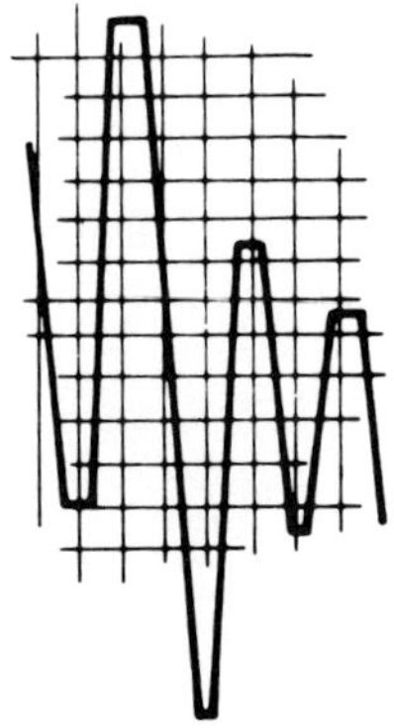

An Assessment of the Contributions

From the Tenth Annual Meeting of the
Society for Advanced Medical Systems (SAMS)
held in Atlanta, Georgia

ADVANCED MEDICAL SYSTEMS:

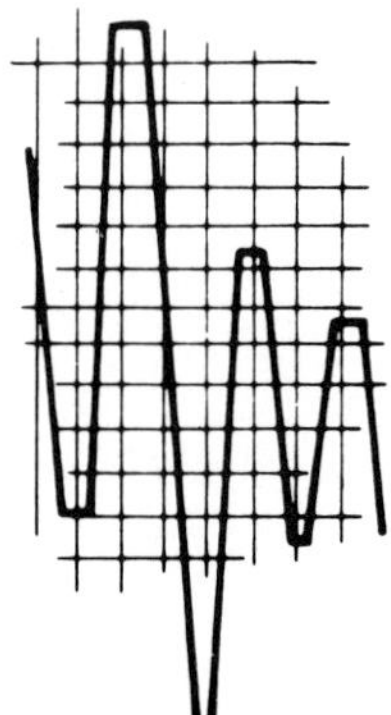

An Assessment of the Contributions

EDWARD J. HINMAN, M.D., M.P.H.
Editor

Executive Director
Group Health Association, Inc.
Washington, D.C.

Published by

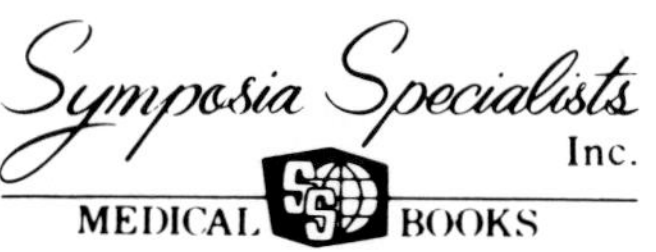

Distributed by

YEAR BOOK
MEDICAL PUBLISHERS
CHICAGO • LONDON

Symposia Specialists, Inc.
1470 N.E. 129th Street
Miami, FL 33161

Distributed by
Year Book Medical Publishers
35 E. Wacker Drive
Chicago, IL 60601

Library of Congress Catalog Card Number 79-66566
International Standard Book Number 0-8151-4460-1

Printed in the United States of America

Contents

Foreword

Since the founding of the Society for Advanced Medical Systems (SAMS) in 1969, the central theme of its annual conference has been continuously changing. The great strength of the Society is that it has been able to provide a common ground of communications for all professionals interested in health care; it is true that at times some may look back to the era of automated multiphasic health testing as the Golden Age of the Society. The Tenth Annual Conference addressed the issue of Advanced Medical Systems: An Assessment of the Contribution. Over 40 professional papers were presented at that conference and enthusiastically received by the participants. Dr. Edward J. Hinman, a past president and now Board member of SAMS, agreed to be the permanent Editor of the Proceedings beginning with this volume. The limited size of the Proceedings does not permit a complete reproduction of all oral communications at the annual conference. Contents of this volume represent a coherent set of quality papers so that the range of communication may be widened.

Richard K. C. Hsieh
President, Society for Advanced Medical Systems
1978 Conference Chairman

Preface

The aims of the Society for Advanced Medical Systems, which was founded in 1969, are to bring together medical personnel, physical scientists, engineers and others to foster cooperation in advancing technology for medical care; to develop standards, terminology and guidelines for the evolution and employment of technological systems which best serve health measurement functions and therapy; to stimulate, sponsor or conduct research in the application and evaluation of technologic systems for detection and treatment of disease states; to promote training and development of professional and allied health manpower needed for advanced medical systems; and to assist in the integration of advanced technological health care systems into the practice of medicine while maintaining high standards of professional ethics.

In October 1978, the 10th Annual Conference was held in Atlanta, Georgia, in conjunction with the 31st Annual Conference on Engineering in Medicine and Biology.

A number of significant papers were presented at this conference. Authors were given the opportunity to submit manuscripts for consideration for publication. An editorial review group to select papers for publication was established by the Society's Board of Directors. This group consisted of Rudolph Bickel, Gilbeart Collings, Harry Emlet, Richard K.C. Hsieh and Edward J. Hinman, as Chief Editor. The papers contained in this volume represent those selected. A diversity of system approaches to health care delivery are addressed. Quality of care, planning and regulations are covered by a number of authors. An update of two multiphasic health testing experiences is also included. The final chapter is a history of the first ten years of the Society.

Readers are encouraged to correspond with authors to continue the dialogue initiated in Atlanta. Interested health care professionals are invited to participate in the 11th Annual Conference to be held October 1979 in Denver.

Special thanks are due to Patricia Horner, Executive Director, and Susan Fletcher, Staff Assistant, for their continued support of SAMS and its Annual Conference.

Edward J. Hinman, M.D., M.P.H.

A Systems Approach to Health

Harry E. Emlet, Jr.

Introduction

Health is a sine qua non of meaningful life. What constitutes meaningful life is judgmental and varies from person to person. While a fully meaningful life may not require full health, clearly some degree of health must exist; in general, the greater the degree of health, the larger the set of options open to the individual to achieve meaningful life.

I define full health for the purpose of this discussion as composed of three elements: absence of disease; existence of full function — physical, mental, and social; and conscious possession of a full sense of well-being. The extent to which all three of these elements are present determines, in large part, the degrees of achievement that are possible for the individual in almost all spheres of life.

In view of this fundamental role of health in human life and achievements, one might expect to find health one of our society's most rational and systematic pursuits. Instead, in the United States today, despite substantial progress over the last several decades in some areas [1], we still find the pursuit of health, in some respects, one of our most haphazard, fragmented and unsystematic activities. If we were to decide to reverse this situation and adopt instead a systems approach to preserving and achieving health and extending meaningful life, how might we proceed? At the conceptual level the basic steps are (1) clearly defining the objectives; (2) identifying the alternative ways of achieving the objectives; (3) selecting the preferred alternative or mix; and (4) implementing the selection. In the case of an ongoing, dynamic process, such as the

---

Harry E. Emlet, Jr., Vice President-Health Systems, ANSER, Arlington, Va.

pursuit of health, these steps are not accomplished once and for all. The process is iterative. The alternatives change with time. The best alternative or mix for achieving the objectives changes with time. The nature and extent of the alternatives from which we can select at any given time are partially governed by the extent to which potential future alternatives were previously recognized and realization of their potential was pursued. That pursuit, when deliberate and systematic, we call research and development (R&D). Thus, the overall system concept must have an important R&D dimension and the steps in the inherent logic become the seven shown in Figure 1. In the remainder of this paper I will briefly consider what is involved in each of these.

Defining the Objectives

The chief objectives in a systems approach to health have already been implicitly or explicitly introduced in the foregoing discussion. As previously stated, the fundamental objective is to achieve and/or preserve health and thereby extend meaningful life. The three components of health — absence of disease, presence of full function and existence of a full sense of well-being — are first-order subobjectives. Those subobjectives stated more fully are: (1) to prevent and, where prevention fails, to control and cure physical and mental disease; (2) to

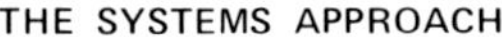

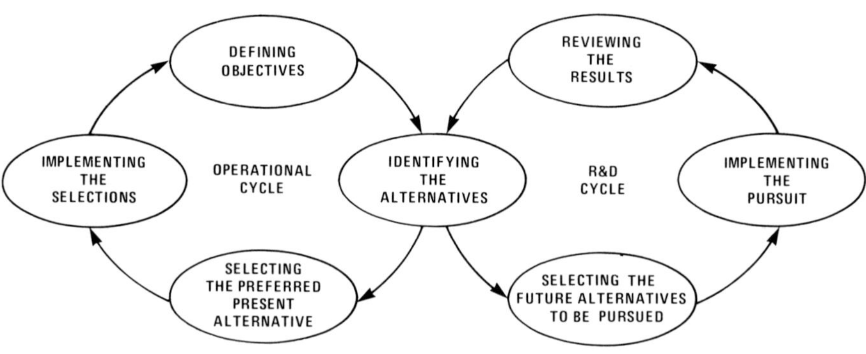

FIGURE 1.

achieve, prevent loss of and, where lost, to restore full physical, mental and social functioning; and (3) to achieve, prevent loss of and, where lost, to restore a full sense of well-being. The third subobjective probably goes well beyond what many if not most health care practitioners would today fully accept as a proper matter of their professional concern. But certainly no one can be considered fully healthy who has a pervading sense that all is not well with him or her. Stating all three objectives in this way implies that some choices have already been made. For example, prevention is a part of each objective, suggesting that simply waiting in all cases until problems develop may not be an acceptable strategy. On the other hand, including prevention as part of the objective does not mean, as we shall soon see, that all possible preventive actions for every potential health problem must be blindly taken. As another example, specifying social functioning — the capacity to interact effectively with other human beings — in the second subobjective suggests that it is as important to health as physical and mental functioning. Of course, it would be possible to consider social functioning as covered under mental functioning, but showing it separately gives it more appropriate emphasis.

Identifying the Alternatives

At the highest level of aggregation, each of the three first-order subobjectives has three potential means of achievement: prevention, early detection and treatment, with or without early detection (Fig. 2). The question is: How and to what extent should each play a role?

For example (Fig. 3), the full set of alternatives to be considered in pursuing the disease-related subobjective through prevention includes three completely different stages of intervention: interventions affecting the prospective parents that occur before the child is conceived; interventions affecting the mother and child that occur after the child is conceived and before he or she is born; and interventions affecting the person after birth. Each stage offers further alternatives for intervention.

For example, in the preconception alternative, at least five suboptions are open. Persons desiring children can select mates

OBJECTIVES
ALTERNATIVES
TO ACHIEVE AND/OR PRESERVE HEALTH AND EXTEND MEANINGFUL LIFE
TO PREVENT AND, WHERE PREVENTION FAILS, CONTROL AND CURE PHYSICAL AND MENTAL DISEASE
TO ACHIEVE, PREVENT LOSS OF, AND, WHERE LOST, RESTORE FULL PHYSICAL, MENTAL, AND SOCIAL FUNCTIONING
TO ACHIEVE, PREVENT LOSS OF, AND, WHERE LOST, RESTORE A FULL SENSE OF WELL–BEING
PREVENTION
EARLY DETECTION
TREATMENT
PREVENTION
EARLY DETECTION
TREATMENT
PREVENTION
EARLY DETECTION
TREATMENT

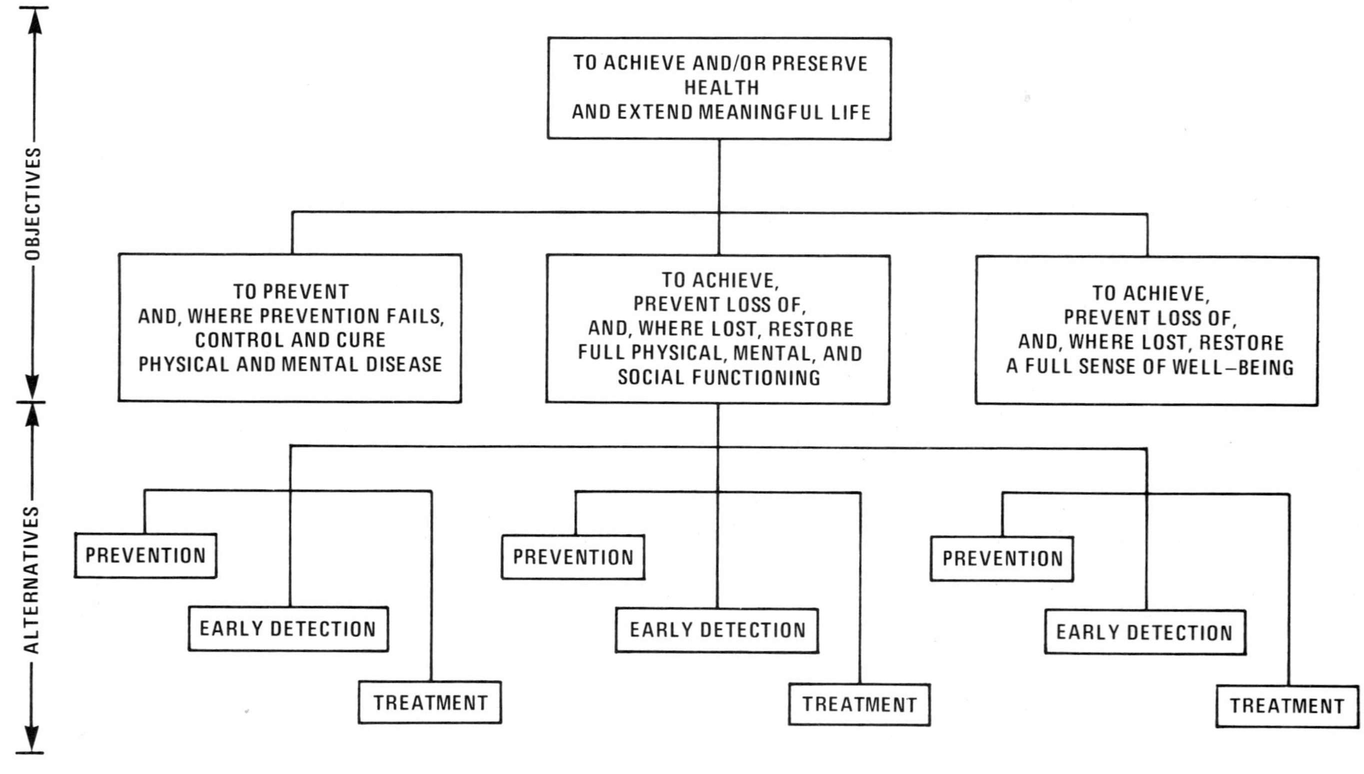

FIGURE 2.

ALTERNATIVES (Continued)
PREVENTION OF DISEASE
PRECONCEPTION
SELECTIVE REPRODUCTION
HEALTH HAZARD AVOIDANCE BY PROSPECTIVE PARENTS
• ENVIRONMENTAL
• PERSONAL PATTERNS OF LIVING
MEDICAL/SURGICAL INTERVENTION
ENVIRONMENTAL CONTROL
GENETIC ENGINEERING
POST–CONCEPTION, PRENATAL
HEALTH HAZARD AVOIDANCE BY MOTHER
• ENVIRONMENTAL
• PERSONAL PATTERNS OF LIVING
MEDICAL/SURGICAL INTERVENTION
ENVIRONMENTAL CONTROL
POST–NATAL
HEALTH HAZARD AVOIDANCE
• ENVIRONMENTAL
• PERSONAL PATTERNS OF LIVING
MEDICAL/SURGICAL INTERVENTION
ENVIRONMENTAL CONTROL

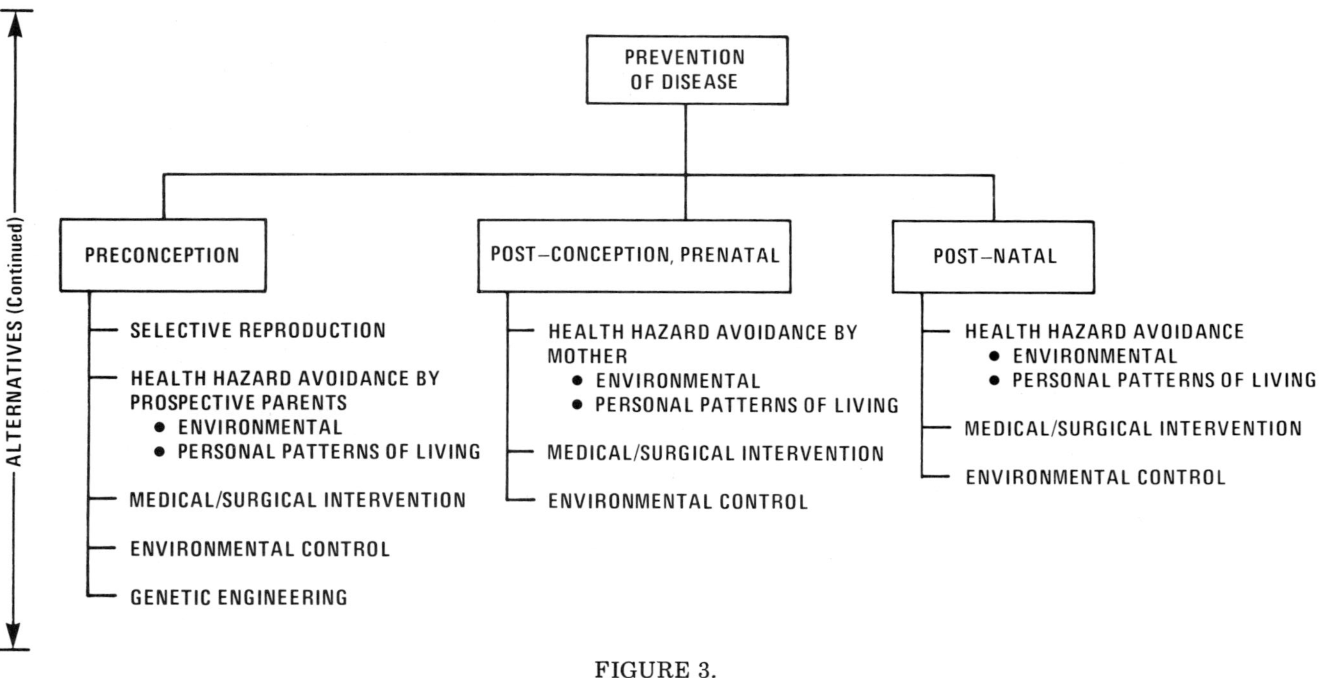

FIGURE 3.

who do not have known genetic factors which would contribute to a likelihood of one or more defects, such as muscular dystrophy; or if already married, they can seek children through adoption rather than reproduction. Health hazards that could affect an as yet unconceived child can be reduced by avoiding either environments or patterns of living which produce them. Diseases, such as syphilis, that could be transmitted to a fetus at or after conception and are of a form and at a stage that is curable can be eliminated by medical or surgical (as appropriate) intervention prior to conception. Factors in the environment prior to conception which would result in deteriorated health in the mother, which persists during pregnancy and affects the fetus, can be eliminated by removing the causative substances from the work environment. Finally, a more futuristic possibility lies in the prospect for actually altering genetic characteristics of a living individual. The middle three of these five alternatives also apply, in somewhat different ways, in both the postconception and postnatal stages.

Each of these alternatives, in turn, represents a large set of more specific kinds of intervention. For example, prevention of disease in the postnatal stage through control or elimination of causal factors in the environment offers a variety of areas of possible intervention, including the atmosphere, water, earth, food, wastes, transportation, shelter, work space factors, recreational space factors and factors in the social milieu, such as those contributing to stress or the lack of a supportive work environment.

Thus far, in the interest of brevity and convenience, I have discussed the consideration of care alternatives (alternative interventions) in a systems approach to health at a level of abstraction that has not considered individual health problems. In practice, if we are to make selections among the intervention alternatives, they must be considered in relation to specific health problems. This consideration imposes, between the objectives levels and the alternatives levels of Figure 2, a health-problem level or levels, as illustrated in Figure 4.

The alternatives I have considered thus far are various kinds of interventions. However, in order for an intervention to occur there must be an organization of resources to make the care available and accessible to the population needing it in form,

TO ACHIEVE AND/OR PRESERVE HEALTH AND EXTEND MEANINGFUL LIFE
TO PREVENT AND, WHERE PREVENTION FAILS, CONTROL AND CURE PHYSICAL AND MENTAL DISEASE
TO ACHIEVE, PREVENT LOSS OF, AND, WHERE LOST, RESTORE FULL PHYSICAL, MENTAL, AND SOCIAL FUNCTIONING
TO ACHIEVE, PREVENT LOSS OF, AND, WHERE LOST, RESTORE A FULL SENSE OF WELL-BEING
VIRAL PNEUMONIA
DIABETES MELLITUS
SCHIZOPHRENIA
LOSS OF HIP FUNCTION
SUBNORMAL LUNG CAPACITY
INABILITY TO CONCENTRATE
INABILITY TO COMMUNICATE
TENSENESS
IRRITABILITY
FEELINGS OF WORTHLESSNESS
PREVENTION
EARLY DETECTION
TREATMENT
OBJECTIVES
HEALTH PROBLEMS
ALTERNATIVES

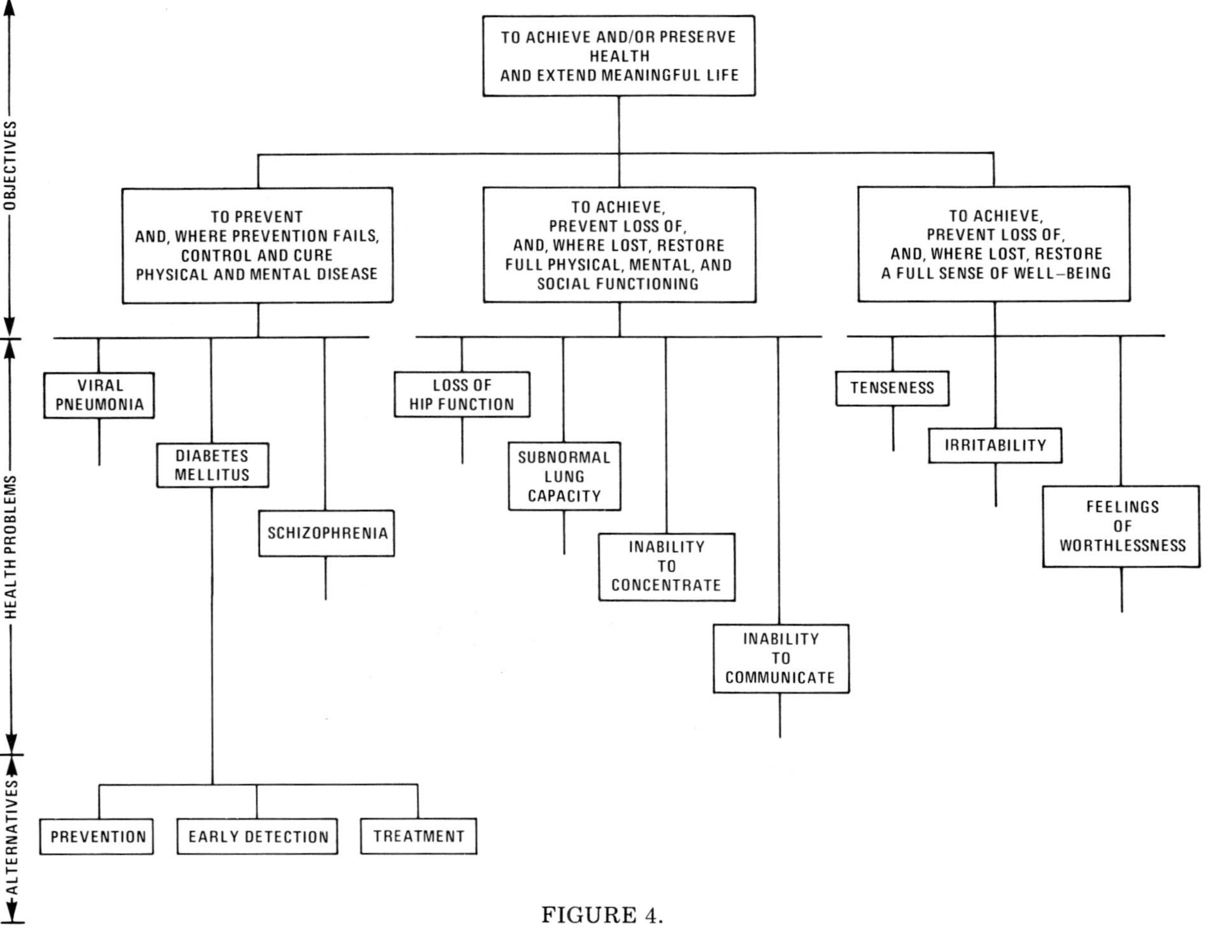

FIGURE 4.

content, quality and costs that make it acceptable to both the patient and the provider and that assure a reasonable likelihood of the patient's realizing the promised benefits. This means that in addition to the intervention options, we must consider organizational options. The organizational design forms the practical context for accomplishing any given set of interventions. Thus, the design of a health care delivery system involves the selection from a variety of both intervention and organizational alternatives. The design is the result of answering a large number of questions either deliberately and explicitly or implicitly by default. Key among these questions are those associated with the items listed around the diagram in Figure 5. For example, what elements (of Figures 2 and 3) are to be included as formal parts of the care system? What are the entry point(s) initially and for each episode (by kind)? Who is responsible for assuring continuity of care? What kind of consumer education exists (by element of care)? What is the basis of selection of persons receiving professional and allied-health-personnel education/training (by personnel category)? How is the technology to be used determined? What method is used to assure quality? Who pays for care?

The answer to each of the main questions associated with each of the 32 items listed in Figure 6 determines an important aspect of the health system design. Each main question clearly has two or more alternative answers. The list is long and, while I believe it includes most of the primary considerations in designing a health care system, it is not exhaustive. I include it to emphasize the point that designing a health care system is a complex process requiring many important decisions.

Selecting the Preferred Present Alternatives

The process of selection that occurs in answering these questions defines the organizational framework within which the full range of health care actions — prevention, early detection and treatment — takes place. The questions are shown in Figure 5 in relation to the general health system design criteria to which each primarily applies. The major criteria are:

1. Availability — does the care component exist?

2. Accessibility — to what extent is the care available in forms, in quantities, at times, at places and at costs that make it possible for the consumer to obtain it when needed?

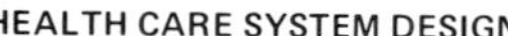

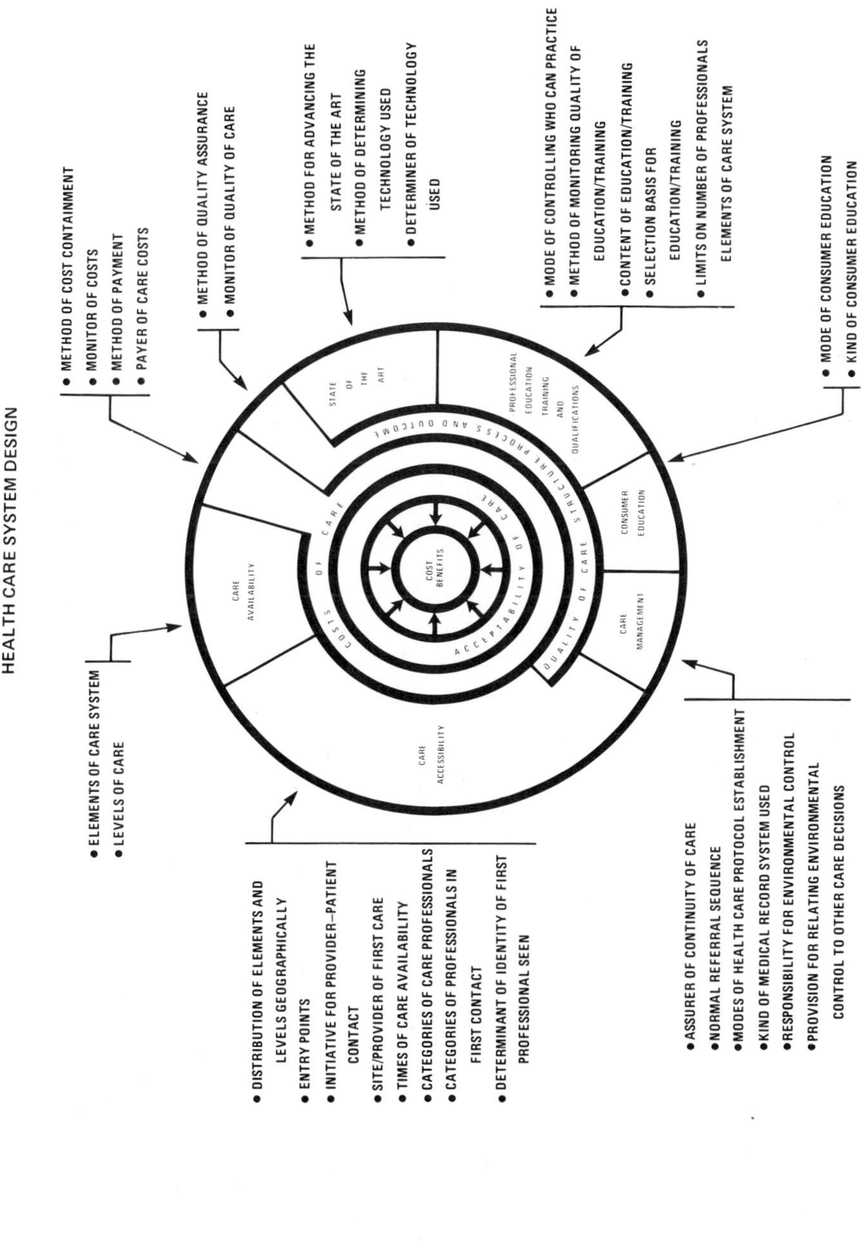

- ELEMENTS OF CARE SYSTEM
- LEVELS OF CARE

- METHOD OF COST CONTAINMENT
- MONITOR OF COSTS
- METHOD OF PAYMENT
- PAYER OF CARE COSTS

- METHOD OF QUALITY ASSURANCE
- MONITOR OF QUALITY OF CARE

- DISTRIBUTION OF ELEMENTS AND LEVELS GEOGRAPHICALLY
- ENTRY POINTS
- INITIATIVE FOR PROVIDER–PATIENT CONTACT
- SITE/PROVIDER OF FIRST CARE
- TIMES OF CARE AVAILABILITY
- CATEGORIES OF CARE PROFESSIONALS
- CATEGORIES OF PROFESSIONALS IN FIRST CONTACT
- DETERMINANT OF IDENTITY OF FIRST PROFESSIONAL SEEN

- METHOD FOR ADVANCING THE STATE OF THE ART
- METHOD OF DETERMINING TECHNOLOGY USED
- DETERMINER OF TECHNOLOGY USED

CARE AVAILABILITY
CARE ACCESSIBILITY
STATE OF THE ART
PROFESSIONAL EDUCATION TRAINING AND QUALIFICATIONS
CONSUMER EDUCATION
CARE MANAGEMENT
COSTS OF CARE
PROCESS AND OUTCOME
QUALITY OF CARE STRUCTURE
ACCEPTABILITY OF CARE
COST BENEFITS

- MODE OF CONTROLLING WHO CAN PRACTICE
- METHOD OF MONITORING QUALITY OF EDUCATION/TRAINING
- CONTENT OF EDUCATION/TRAINING
- SELECTION BASIS FOR EDUCATION/TRAINING
- LIMITS ON NUMBER OF PROFESSIONALS ELEMENTS OF CARE SYSTEM

- ASSURER OF CONTINUITY OF CARE
- NORMAL REFERRAL SEQUENCE
- MODES OF HEALTH CARE PROTOCOL ESTABLISHMENT
- KIND OF MEDICAL RECORD SYSTEM USED
- RESPONSIBILITY FOR ENVIRONMENTAL CONTROL
- PROVISION FOR RELATING ENVIRONMENTAL CONTROL TO OTHER CARE DECISIONS

- MODE OF CONSUMER EDUCATION
- KIND OF CONSUMER EDUCATION

FIGURE 5.

SIMPLIFIED SCHEMATIC OF PROPOSED APPROACH TO MODELING BENEFITS OF ALTERNATIVE CARE PROGRAMS

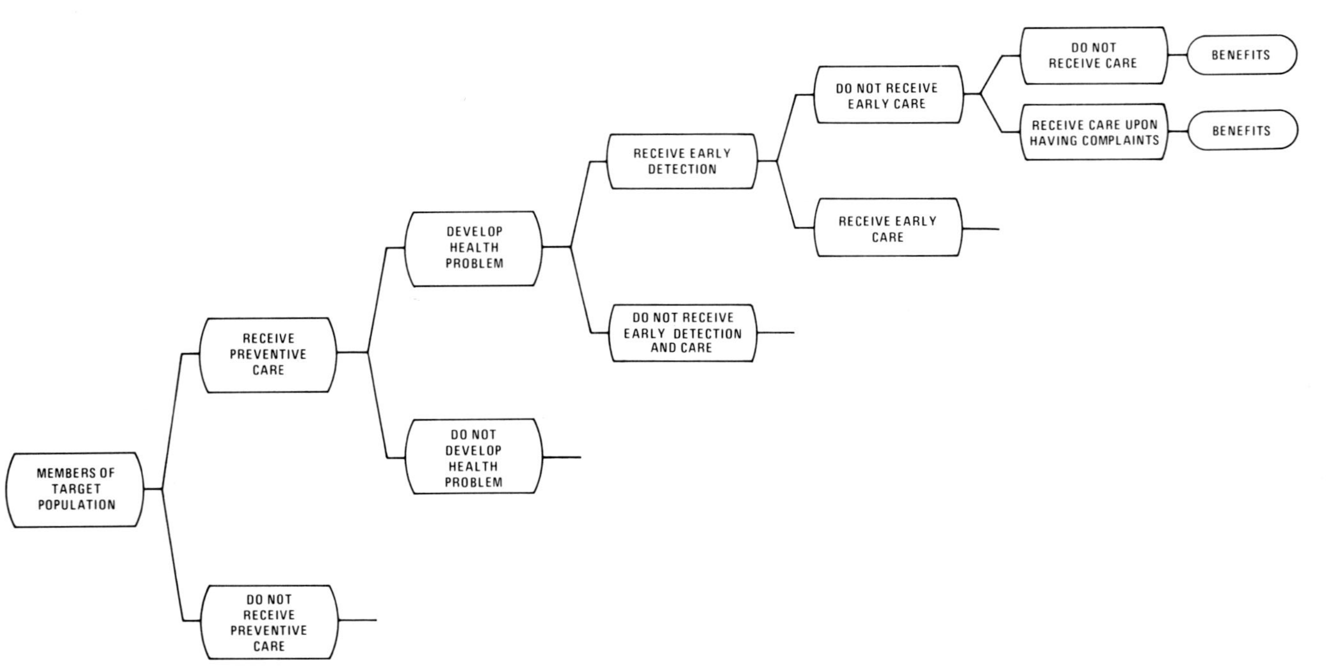

FIGURE 6.

3. Quality — to what extent does the care provided meet established standards in terms of structure, process and health outcomes? (Major categories of specific criteria affecting quality are care management policies and practices, consumer health-educational level attained, provider health-educational level attained, and state-of-the-art of care methods and means.)

4. Cost — what are the costs of providing and applying the resources within the organizational framework selected? These costs both influence and are influenced by how and to what extent the other criteria mentioned thus far are met.

5. Acceptability — to what extent is the care — as it is available and accessible and, in view of its quality and costs — also acceptable to consumer, provider and payer? Acceptability is a function of the extent to which all the previous criteria are met.

The criterion which conceptually ties all of these other criteria together is the cost-benefit criterion: what combination of interventions and organizational options provides the greatest cost-benefits within the resources available? The end benefits are the health outcomes measured in terms of health status. The intermediate benefits are many, including the degrees of availability, accessibility and quality (in terms of structure and process) that are attained.

While, conceptually, the cost-benefit criterion ties all of the other criteria together, in actual practice the evaluation task is made more complex by the fact that there is no single measure of overall cost-benefits [2]. Some of the benefits are dollar benefits; some are translatable into dollars; but others defy translation into dollars. Some benefits cannot be quantified in even non-dollar units. What we can do is evaluate all those benefits and costs that can be quantified; sum those quantifiable in dollars (present value); sum by common units and list those benefits quantifiable in non-dollar units, such as extended years of life and reduced days bedridden; and list the remaining purely qualitative benefits. When similar summaries of dollar cost-benefits and non-dollar benefits have been made for each alternative, then a judgment must be made as to which alternative yields on balance the greatest cost-benefits. This kind of analysis can be very helpful in sorting out the relative merits of alternative courses of action, and any serious pursuits of a systems approach to health will use such analyses extensively. The author and his colleagues are successfully applying this analytic approach to assist in decisions on major health systems equipment procurements [3-5].

In exploring the benefits of alternative programs of intervention where each program offers a somewhat different mix of prevention, early detection and treatment, we would like for example to undertake for each health problem an analysis of the form suggested in Figure 6 — an analysis that a colleague* and I proposed to HEW in 1972. For each given health problem, each person in a population follows one and only one path in a lifetime. The model can be designed to calculate for a given health problem the benefits to be expected for the population, given estimates of (1) the probability for each event in the path that a person in each cohort considered will experience that event and (2) the benefit that the person who completes the path would realize. A complementary cost model can be developed which will calculate the total costs for the population, given estimates of costs associated with each event for a person in each cohort and for each organization alternative that is considered as a possible context for delivering the given program of intervention. Thus, the cost-benefits of each alternative health care system design can be calculated.

Implementing such a model is a sizable task. However, it can be done at many different levels of detail. At the present level of the state-of-the-art of such modeling and the knowledge of the probabilities and benefits associated with each path and cohort, it would be wise to explore the results at higher levels of aggregation, proceeding to the next level of greater detail only as experience is gained and useful results are obtained at the previous level.

Since much of the hard data needed for such analysis does not now exist, conduct of the analysis is dependent upon extensive use of estimates by experts. That experts can agree on estimates of the kinds of probabilities and benefits required for such a model was established by the author and his colleagues in a 1973 study of post-onset care for stroke [6]. Preliminary evidence of good correlations between the estimates of that

*John L. Davis, Ph.D., ANSER.

study and actual experience has since been reported in a study at Hennipen General Hospital in Minneapolis [7]. The results of the initial study [6] showed very different cost-benefits for alternative modes of care for stroke for different patient groups, as illustrated by the sample of the results shown in Figure 7.

Selecting the Future Alternatives To Be Pursued

At the level of detail of the alternative interventions shown in Figure 3, each alternative has under it more specific alternatives, some of which are now feasible technically and operationally, with the exception of genetic engineering where the investigators are still probing the threshold. The more specific alternatives have among them a wide range of technical and operational feasibility. If we are to apply the systems approach to the future alternatives, we must begin by distinguishing the existing stage of development of each alternative (at the final level of specificity) and the stages remaining before each can reach full operational status. At each stage a different set of actions or activities is appropriate. Figure 8 lists the stages

COST–BENEFITS OF POST–ONSET CARE FOR STROKE
(ESTIMATED INCREASE IN DAYS WITH
LESS IMPAIRMENT THAN WHEN REQUIRING SUPERVISION
PER THOUSAND DOLLARS OF CARE COSTS)

	CARE RULE	
PATIENT–GROUP A	OPTIMUM	2.4
	AVERAGE	0
PATIENT–GROUP B	OPTIMUM	74.8
	AVERAGE	17.1
PATIENT–GROUP C	OPTIMUM	288
	AVERAGE	318
PATIENT–GROUP D	OPTIMUM	128
	AVERAGE	32

FIGURE 7.

FEASIBILITY STAGES AND APPROPRIATE R&D ACTIONS

FEASIBILITY STAGE	APPROPRIATE ACTION
PRECONCEPTUAL	PROBLEM DEFINITION CONCEPTUALIZATION STUDIES
CONCEPTUAL	CONCEPT ANALYSIS AND EVALUATION BASIC RESEARCH
SCIENTIFICALLY VALID	EXPLORATORY DEVELOPMENT
TECHNICALLY FEASIBLE	ADVANCED DEVELOPMENT
PRODUCIBLE AND OPERATIONALLY FEASIBLE	ENGINEERING DEVELOPMENT OPERATIONAL DEVELOPMENT OPERATIONAL DEMONSTRATION AND EVALUATION
OPERATIONAL	OPERATION CONTINUING EVALUATION PROCESS OUTCOME COST–BENEFIT

FIGURE 8.

in ascending order of the feasibility that has been established and shows the kind of R&D action that is appropriate for the indicated stages if resources are to be invested to attempt to advance the potential alternative to the next stage of feasibility [8].

The criteria for evaluating the potential future alternatives are the same as for present alternatives. However, the following several new factors are very important in assessing the cost-benefits of the alternatives and in selecting from among them:

1. R&D costs.
2. Likelihood of successfully concluding the final stage.
3. Confidence limits on the expected benefits and the estimated costs of achieving them.

The importance of the first two factors can be seen by an examination of the illustration of Figure 9. In general, as a future alternative progresses through the sequence from concept to full operational status, our ability improves to forecast the likelihood of its proceeding to the final stage and the cost increases of advancing it to the next appropriate stage (although, not every newly conceived alternative that eventually reaches the last stage need pass through all the intermediate stages).

Figure 9 compares with the present mode of care (the first column) three different hypothetical future options (the next three columns), each requiring R&D. The figure first compares the options in terms of health benefits only (with the measure being extended years of life) and then successively in terms of research cost, cost-benefits of research, other R&D costs, two kinds of operating costs, total costs, total cost-benefits, probability of success of several stages in the basic research-to-operating-system sequence and, finally, expected benefits and expected cost-benefits. The main points to be noted are that (1) while the third alternative starts out the clear winner by an enormous margin, as additional cost and risk considerations are introduced, its lead is progressively narrowed until it loses decisively to the second alternative; (2) the first alternative never gets into the running on either benefits or cost-benefits, despite the fact that it has a clear edge on over half of the contributing values; (3) the expected cost-benefits of the winner are more than 26 times those of the poorest alternative; and

COMPARISON OF ALTERNATIVES*
IN TERMS OF BENEFITS, COSTS,
COST–BENEFITS, EXPECTED BENEFITS,
AND EXPECTED COST–BENEFITS†

		ALTERNATIVES			
		—	1	2	3
BENEFITS (K YEARS)		27.6	110.6	414.7	**4,052.8**
COST OF RESEARCH ($M)		0	**0.2**	1.0	2.0
COST–BENEFITS OF RESEARCH (YRS/$K)†		∞	553.0	414.7	**2,026.4**
COST ($M)	COMPLEMENTARY AND FOLLOWUP R&D	0	**0.2**	5.0	10.0
	SCREENING	0	120.0	**0**	**0**
	CARE	94.6	378.2	**13.5**	129.5
	TOTAL	94.6	498.6	**19.5**	141.5
COST–BENEFITS, TOTAL (YRS/$K)		0.3	0.2	21.3	**28.6**
PROBABILITY OF SUCCESS	RESEARCH	—	**0.6**	0.5	0.3
	FOLLOWUP R&D	—	**0.8**	0.7	0.6
	COMPLEMENTARY R&D	—	**1.0**	0.5	0.2
	ACCEPTANCE	—	**0.9**	0.7	0.8
	OPERATIONAL	—	**0.9**	0.8	0.8
	OVERALL	—	**0.389**	0.098	0.023
EXPECTED	BENEFITS (K YEARS)	27.6	43.0	40.6	**93.2**
	COST–BENEFITS, TOTAL (YRS/$K)	0.3	0.08	**2.1**	0.66

*SHADED VALUES HIGHLIGHT THE BEST VALUE ON EACH MEASURE
†BENEFITS ARE IN YEARS OF EXTENDED LIFE

FIGURE 9.

(4) these results become apparent only if you take the trouble to work through the calculations.

The illustration does not show the possible effect of considering the confidence limits on each of the contributing values. (These limits are the end points of the range of values within which there is believed to be a high probability, e.g., .95, that the true value lies.) However, it is clear that if the confidence limits were narrow for all three R&D options, the results would not change. If the confidence limits were very different for each of the three, the winner could change. If the confidence limits were wide on all three, the result could be that there is no clear winner.

An important message from the considerations of the preceding paragraphs is that a systems approach to pursuit of future alternatives may greatly increase the effectiveness of the R&D dollars spent.

Implementing the Preferred Course of Action

In the case of either a preferred present alternative or a preferred future alternative to be pursued through R&D, the systems approach in the implementation phase is basically the same:

1. Carefully map out the implementation plan.
2. Closely monitor and control the implementation to assure that it follows the plan.
3. Continually evaluate the results to insure that the expected benefits and cost-benefits are being realized.
4. Modify the plan and its implementation as the results of the evaluation and associated considerations indicate appropriate.

This sequence of steps provides for feedback and control which is found infrequently today in the implementation of health care system innovations and which is almost essential to insure that innovations lead to improved health care delivery and health and not simply oscillations about the status quo or, worse, steady deterioration.

Conclusion

Application of the systems approach to health requires a deliberate and comprehensive identification and assessment of all the alternative paths to achieving and preserving health. Some of the alternatives, such as prevention through control of the environment, fall outside of what is now considered the primary purview of health care; and yet they may represent the most powerful and cost-effective way of influencing certain aspects of health. Other alternatives involve educating the consumer and bringing him into a role in caring for his or her health that goes well beyond what health care providers are now prepared to do or accept and may well entail enlisting the direct involvement of the public and private school systems.

Still other alternatives, such as those related to achieving and maintaining a full sense of well-being, require the health care provider to assume responsibility for an area he is untrained or ill-trained to understand and address and that he tends to regard as involving largely "personal problems" of minor significance in comparison with disease and clearly identifiable loss of function. Addressing this category of system concern may require significantly revising the content of medical education and the criteria for selection of its recipients or, alternatively, the development of an entirely new kind of health care provider, the educational framework to educate and train him or her and the organizational setting in which he or she is to function. Yet another direction is conceptualization, exploration and development of entirely new paths, such as genetic engineering, which may hold the key to a breakthrough in some chronic health problems similar to what antibiotics provided for infectious disease.

If the systems approach is seriously adopted, these areas outside the normal scope of health care are not simply noted and dismissed as options someone else should do something about, but are deliberately addressed as alternatives; analyzed and evaluated to determine their relative significance; and, if shown to be sufficiently significant, implemented in a manner appropriate to their stage and role in the overall system.

Certainly, one of the first steps in such a systems approach is to identify at the national level who has or should have the necessary comprehensive cognizance and authority for initiating the systems planning, recommending the system-wide courses of action and implementing or securing implementation of the recommendations. A next large step is to accomplish the planning necessary to identify a rational, systematic course of action. The next large step after that is to provide and apply the resources required to implement the plan.

References

1. Hinman, E.J.: Advanced medical systems: Progress, prospects and challenges. *In* Emlet, Jr., H.E.: Challenges and Prospects for Advanced Medical Systems. Miami, Fla.:Symposia Specialists, 1978, pp. 1-10.

2. Emlet, Jr., H.E., Carlisle, R.G. et al: Measures and Indicators for Evaluation of Innovations to the Health Care System. HSDN 77-2, Analytic Services Inc., June 1977.
3. Brooks, R.C., Casey, I.J. and Blackmon, Jr., P.W.: Evaluation of the Air Force Clinical Laboratory Automation System (AFCLAS) at Wright-Patterson USAF Medical Center. Volume I, Summary. HSDN 77-4, Analytic Services Inc., January 1977 (updated May 1977), pp. 42, NTIS No. AD-A043 664.
4. Brooks, R.C., Casey, I.J. and Blackmon, Jr., P.W.: Evaluation of the Air Force Clinical Laboratory Automation System (AFCLAS). Volume II, Analysis. HSDN 77-5, Analytic Services Inc., May 1977, pp. 354, NTIS No. AD-A043 665.
6. Emlet, Jr., H.E., Williamson, J.W., Dittmer, D.L. and Davis, J.L.: Estimated Health Benefits and Costs of Post-Onset Care for Stroke. Report prepared by Analytic Services Inc. in cooperation with and under subcontract to The Johns Hopkins University and in cooperation with InterStudy, American Rehabilitation Foundation under grants from the Department of Health, Education and Welfare, September 1973.
7. Anderson, T.P., Baldridge, M. and Ettinger, M.G.: Quality of Care for Completed Stroke Without Rehabilitation: Evaluation by Assessing Patient Outcomes. Presented at 1976 American Congress of Rehabilitation Medicine and accepted for publication in the Archives of Physical Medicine.
8. Emlet, Jr., H.E.: Economic analysis of health programs. *In* Planning Biomedical Research Programs. (U.S. DHEW, NIH, National Cancer Institute, February 1974), pp. 5-1 to 5-30.

Assessment of Quality Review in the Health Care System: The Hospital

William H. Forrest, Jr., M.D.

When approaching this problem of quality review, perhaps our first question should be: "Why bother? Its very costly to do!" I don't think it is within my charge here to address that important question, so I will assume that the answer is either (1) we should do it even if it is not cost effective or (2) we have to develop a system of quality review which is cost effective.

Why hospitals? Why should we focus our attention on inpatient short-term care? Short-term hospitals are clearly a principal segment of the health care system. Slightly greater than one out of every 10 persons in the United States is hospitalized in this type of facility each year [1], and hospital care is the largest expenditure category in national health care spending (approximately 40%). There are about 7,450 hospitals in the United States of which approximately 87% are general medical and surgical hospitals.

Short-term hospitals are defined as facilities having six beds or more for inpatient use and a mean length of stay of 30 days or less. In this component of the total health care system we are probably dealing with 32 million discharges annually and 250 million patient days of care. I think you would agree the system is large enough to justify its due place for quality assessment . . . but does it need to be assessed?

Is there a problem in quality? There are a multitude of answers to that question and they vary from the extreme of categorically no to a qualified yes. The consensus, however, is

---

William H. Forrest, Jr., M.D., Department of Anesthesia, Stanford University School of Medicine, Stanford, Calif.

yes and it comes from the many articles which chronicle deficiencies in the provision of hospital-based care. A few examples: Fine and Morehead [2] reported deficiencies in care process in cases of appendectomy, hysterectomy and prostatectomy in six New York hospitals; Helbig et al [3], using a care component score to study the care for handicapped children, reported considerable incompleteness in diagnostic work-up.

In my own studies at Stanford Center for Health Care Research [4] we demonstrated a threefold difference in expected outcomes for selected surgical procedures among 17 short stay hospitals. The quality of care criteria were post-operative deaths and morbidity carefully controlled for patient mix. We do not know whether we can influence permanent change, but we have demonstrated differences. Thus, for both process and outcome of care substantial differences in care quality exist.

Given these differences in quality, what are we doing to assess and minimize them? It is safe to say we are expending enormous energy to try to effect change and we really do not know how well we are doing. Using methods espoused by JCAH and PSRO or combinations of these and other approaches, almost all, if not all, hospitals review the care delivered. The major thrusts of these evaluation schemes are to establish norms of care (standards), look for deficiencies either retrospectively or concurrently and effect improvement by decreasing or eliminating these deficiencies. Over the last few years more and more emphasis has been placed on evaluating the outcomes of care. However, little is known about how well we are doing, that is, the outcomes of our quality assessments.

Jesse [5] outlined his assessment of how we are doing. His mostly philosophical but probably fair evaluation is as follows:

1. Assessment suffers from stereotyped approaches and technical ineptitude.
2. Topic selection is divorced from monitoring data and other systems which identify problems.
3. Criteria are often imprecise, exceptionally complex and unrelated to the audit topic.
4. Variation (deficiency) analysis focuses on justification of individual cases rather than looking for patterns of care.

Thus, he feels the present system has severe limitations.

Sanazaro [6] recently reported a study of 5,604 cases in 50 hospitals belonging to several PSROs, comparing concurrent monitoring to retrospective monitoring in several diagnostic categories. It is noteworthy that there was a 1% difference in adherence to criteria and a 4% difference in documentation favoring the group which utilized concurrent review. He also confirmed the existence of substantial differences among hospitals in the proportion of patients experiencing preventable complications. Direct cost to the patients for the quality assessment was $1.23 per day for data collection (no figures were given for data processing). Sanazaro's data provide us with some of the essential elements which are necessary to calculate the cost-benefit of quality assessment, but only give us beginning information on our ability to effect permanent change.

Jesse [5] comments that for the most part, corrective action depends upon written directives — ignoring well-established principles of individual and organizational behavior. He notes that most hospitals have audits, but few have succeeded in obtaining lasting change. Hospitals are complex organizations with overlapping responsibilities shared by boards of directors, medical staffs and administrators. There are diverse goals, diffuse authority, low task interdependence and few performance measures. All these factors make change difficult.

Jesse does recommend (1) scientific evaluation of quality assessment schemes; (2) better understanding of process and outcome; (3) improved external monitoring; and (4) increased public awareness.

In a recent analysis of the issues in health care evaluation, McDermott [7] concluded that "the concepts on which the present quality assurance movement is based are unproved propositions. Even if some of these concepts do prove to be valid, we can still recognize potentially serious pitfalls in the current programs which could actually lower the quality of care in some institutions or areas of the country, or could raise costs of care without providing compensating gains in quality [8]." A critical shortcoming which has not been adequately stressed is that there are no quantitative goals against which to measure performance. PSRO and JCAH may set goals "but the goals are not expressed in terms that might permit measurement of the degree to which they are achieved" [9].

A system based on our work could overcome many of these critical defects. Using patient abstract data, the system would monitor all short-term hospitals for utilization of services and outcome of care and, most importantly, it would reserve the very expensive intensive inhouse audit systems, such as those now proliferating (PSRO and JCAH), for those hospitals identified by this monitoring system as relatively ineffective in delivering health care — hospitals where the biggest improvement could be expected, so the effort would be cost-effective. The system is designed to measure the effect of services provided and the quality of outcomes and would monitor the impact of cost-containment measures on both cost and quality of care. The system would be ongoing, allowing measurement of changes over time.

The program proposed deals with important dimensions of care which can be measured simply and economically and which can be expected to yield to efforts at improvement. This would be in distinct contrast to the more intensive, comprehensive and very costly attempts to contain costs and improve care through JCAH and PSRO review, where the costs are already high, estimated at $10 to $22 per patient discharged and spiraling, with no way of comparing present performance or plans to measure performance trends.

Recent studies [4] by the Stanford Center for Health Care Research have shown that abstracts of patient charts can be used to measure the quality and cost of care in hospitals. These studies involved summary data from the Professional Activity Study (PAS) of the Commission for Professional and Hospital Activities (CPHA). PAS data were compared with date obtained from a more intensive study in a small number of hospitals. The intensive study results were consistent with the outcome evaluations based on PAS information. Our most recent study demonstrated that it is possible to utilize routinely abstracted summary data to distinguish between performance levels in different hospitals in three important ways: (1) on the basis of a single outcome — death in the hospital; (2) on the basis of length of stay; and (3) on the basis of intensity of services provided. This differentiation among hospitals is particularly important at the extremes, where ratios of observed performance to expected performance varied significantly and the magnitudes are of national public concern. More importantly, in this study it was possible to examine the relationships between quality and the critically important cost-performance measures, such as intensity of services and length of stay. Details of the methods and results can be found in a series of published reports [4]. An abbreviated summary of the method follows.

PAS abstract information from over 600,000 cases discharged in 1970 to 1973 from 17 randomly selected PAS member hospitals provided the basic data set for the comparison of outcomes, service intensity and length of stay. The 600,000 cases represented virtually all non-newborn discharges from the hospitals (99%). The 17 hospitals were a stratified random sample from approximately 1,200 general short-term PAS hospitals; thus, our findings are extrapolated to this larger set of hospitals.

Selected data from the 80 item PAS Abstract were used to define the outcome variable, Death at Discharge; a process variable, Length of Stay; and a service intensity variable based upon several service measures (such as use of intensive care, blood and drugs administered, x-ray and laboratory tests performed). Other PAS items including Admission Blood Pressure, Pulse, Temperature, Hemoglobin, White Blood Cells, Chronic Diagnoses and certain drugs indicating chronic illness were used in specially prepared algorithms to adjust the dependent variables for varying patient mix in the several hospitals. Finally, hospitals were ranked on the basis of their adjusted death rates, adjusted average lengths of stay and adjusted measures of service intensity.

Results of the analyses were as follows:

1. After carefully adjusting for differences in patient mix, discharge status and complications and correcting for random variation, it was estimated that the 16% of hospitals at the high end of the distribution (one standard deviation above the mean) kept patients on the average of 2.5 days longer than those at the low end (one standard deviation or more, below the mean).

2. After adjusting for patient mix the 16% of hospitals at the high end of the distribution had death rates 80% higher than hospitals at the low end of the distribution.

3. After adjusting for patient mix the 16% of hospitals at the high end of the distribution provided 17% more services than expected, based on all patients in all 17 hospitals.

4. When crude death rates for the hospitals were examined, length of stay appeared to be a weak surrogate for the outcome of death in the hospital, and the effects of hospital services provided to patients were not evident. However, after careful standardization of mortality and length of stay for case mix, length of stay was highly correlated with mortality and an inverse relationship of service intensity to mortality was clear and strong. Thus, shorter stay, higher service intensity and lower mortality were highly associated after adjustment for patient mix in the hospitals.

These results suggest that an abstract system, perhaps the PAS, some minor modification of it, or a similar system could be used on an ongoing basis to monitor the nation's hospitals, and that the hospitals be ranked periodically in the order of their case mix adjusted performance. Potentially useful methods for adjusting the performance measures, death at discharge, length of stay and service intensity have been developed by the Stanford Center for Health Research [4].

Rankings of hospitals based on these adjusted measures would be available to both the provider and consumer. As an important first step the proposed monitoring system could evaluate the effect of release of this ranking information on the important performance measures.

In addition, the data used to rank hospitals would be used to set specific goals for improvement. Hospitals targeted for more intensive onsite audit of the type now promulgated by PSRO and JCAH might be the 16% with the poorest performance for one or more of the performance measures — for example, those with the highest adjusted death rates or the highest adjusted lengths of stay. The overall goals would be to reduce the number of postoperative deaths in these hospitals by some specific amount — perhaps to reduce the adjusted rates for the poorer hospitals to the current national median. Equally important, one could institute rational approaches to cost-containment based on knowledge of the interaction of adjusted length of stay, service intensity and mortality.

The idea of using PAS or similar abstract information as the basis of quality assessment is not new. Slee has outlined a hospital quality control system based on PAS data [10]. McDermott called attention to the comparative operative mortality available with the CPHA Quality Assurance Monitor and suggested that "a properly organized surgical staff" could use this information "to ensure maintenance of quality" [7]. Thus far, however, little progress has been made along these lines. Currently, systems of unproven validity provide information on performance which is not widely disseminated and does not reveal results to other hospitals or the consumer. We believe the time has come to use these data effectively to improve hospital performance when indicated.

Several writers have raised the question of whether efforts at quality assessment and assurance will prove cost-effective [9, 11]. The difference between previous plans and the program proposed is that this program is directed specifically at those hospitals where the greatest improvements could be made with the least investment. It is a well-known principle that the same expenditure will produce different results in different institutions, depending upon the capacity of each institution for improvement. Thus, in hospitals at or near the peak of accomplishment for certain types of operations, only minor improvements in postoperative death rates could be expected, even with large investments of money and effort. Hospitals with mortality two or more times as large as the mean for all hospitals, however, would have much room for improvement, and even a modest investment should create a reasonable payoff.

Recognizing that the wisest investment would be in hospitals where the greatest returns could be expected, one might even elect not to audit high performance hospitals other than by routine monitoring to verify that they have maintained their high ranking. Should new technology better the performance of these institutions, routine screening would detect the change in mortality. This would then provide new performance guidelines for those hospitals not doing as well as the leaders.

It is remarkable that with all the effort that has gone into quality assurance to date, there is still no measurable nationwide goal. Millions of dollars have been invested without specification of a destination. How will we know whether we have arrived at our goal? Are the goals of PSRO to double the quality of care, halve hospital death rates, make the quality even across the country?

The goal of lowering mortality in the 16% of hospitals with the highest mortality is of course not stated precisely enough. Should the rates in those institutions be reduced to the national median? The specific targets should be developed by representatives of the medical profession, government, private third party insurers and consumers. The representatives will have to recognize that the more ambitious the goal, the greater the cost is likely to be. But at least there will be a real target to aim for, a recognizable landmark so the public and the professions will know whether the project has reached its destination.

It is now feasible to measure with a proven methodology the performance of U.S. short-term hospitals. Hospitals identified as having the poorest performances could then be the focus of efforts to improve care. Results are available that suggest the specific form such efforts might take. Continued monitoring and randomized studies of such groups of poor performance hospitals are suggested to validate the efforts and to measure the achievements of the program. The measurements obtained should yield valuable insights into the potential for economical and cost-effective quality assurance programs in the U.S. short-term hospitals.

References

1. The Nations Use of Health Resources. U.S. Department of Health Education and Welfare, 1976, DHEW (HRA) 77-1240.
2. Fine, J. and Morehead, M.A.: Study of peer review of in-hospital patient care. N.Y. State J. Med. 71:1963-1973, 1971.
3. Helbig, D.W., O'Hare, D. and Smith, N.W.: The care component score: A new system for evaluating the quality of inpatient care. Am. J. Public Health 62:540-546, 1972.
4. Stanford Center for Health Care Research:
   a. Comparison of hospitals with regard to outcomes of surgery. Health Services Research, 11 (Summer 1976), 112-127.
   b. Hospital structure and postoperative mortality and morbidity. Preliminary findings from a survey of 17 hospitals. *In* Shortell, S.M. and Brown, M. (eds.): Organizational Research in Hospitals. Chicago:Blue Cross Association, an Inquiry Book, 1976.
   c. Study of the Institutional Differences in Postoperative Mortality: A Report to the National Academy of Sciences, DHEW PB 2500940/LK. Springfield, Va.:National Technical Information Service, December 1974.

d. Studies of Determinants of Service Intensity in the Medical Care Sector. A Final Report to the National Center for Health Services Research, DNEW under Contract HRA 203-75-0169. September 1977.

e. Impact of Hospital Characteristics on Surgical Outcomes and Length of Stay. A final report to the National Center for Health Services Research, DHEW under Contract HRA 230-75-0173, July 1978.

5. Jesse, F.: Quality Assessment Systems—Why aren't there any? Q.R.B. 3(11):16-18, 1977.
6. Sanazaro, P.J.: Concurrent quality assurance in hospital care: Report of a study by a private institution in PSRO. N. Engl. J. Med. 298(21):1171-1177, May 25, 1978.
7. McDermott, W.: Evaluating the physician and his technology. Daedalus, Vol. 106-1, 135-158, 1977.
8. Advancing the Quality of Health Care. Institute of Medicine. National Academy of Sciences. Wash. D.C., August, 1974.
9. Assessing the Quality of Health Care. An Evolution. Institute of Medicine. National Academy of Sciences. Wash., D.C., November 1974.
10. Slee, S.N.: PSRO and the hospital quality control. Ann. Intern. Med. 81:97-106, 1974.
11. Brook, R.H., Williams, K.N. and Avery, A.D.: Quality assurance today and tomorrow: Forecast for the future. Ann. Intern. Med. 85:809-817, 1976.

Assessing the Quality of a Review System for Ambulatory Care

Paul Y. Ertel, M.D. and Inta J. Ertel, M.D.

The quality of any medical review system is measured by the extent to which it brings about desirable change in the delivery of medical care. While this may appear to be self-evident, inexplicably, the practical applications of this fundamental concept are often overlooked. This paper will examine what is involved in assessing the quality of a review system by measuring desirable changes in ambulatory care that are causally related to review activities.

While the focus will be upon theoretical considerations, the presentation will be illustrated by application of basic concepts in a functioning primary child care program.

The unequivocal demonstration of a causal relationship between the introduction of a review system and any changes that may have taken place in the delivery of care is difficult enough. Beyond this, all the inherent problems are compounded when one attempts to take the next logical step which is to ascertain whether any of the observed changes in care that may be attributable to the review system actually constitute *improvements*. This entails another whole set of tasks involved in objectively determining the impact of changes in the care system with respect to an improved health status and well-being of patients (ultimate effects).

Whatever the difficulties in establishing causal relationships and clinical outcomes, they cannot be made any simpler by skipping steps in data acquisition. For example, if there is only an incomplete description of the care system or if its status is

Paul Y. Ertel, M.D. and Inta J. Ertel, M.D., Health Services Research Center and the Pediatric Unit, University Health Plan, The University of Michigan, Ann Arbor.

unknown *prior to* the introduction of the review system, then it will not be possible to determine to what extent or even whether any change at all has been effected by the review system. If there is no accepted concept of what constitutes a "good" care system (i.e., a model), then one cannot judge whether any observed changes are in the right direction (i.e., are "desirable"). If there is no knowledge of the health status of patients prior to and subsequent to the observed changes in the care system initiated by the review system, then there is no way to ascertain whether the health and well-being of patients have been improved. Therefore, we will next consider what kinds of data are needed to adequately describe the quality of medical care being delivered and its impact on patients, plus the kinds of data that are needed to describe the review system itself and its impact upon care delivery. Following these general considerations, we will examine the total data requirements needed to evaluate both the care system and the review system in the ambulatory setting.

Description of the Care System

Donabedian's classic description of the quality of medical care, i.e., his triad consisting of the structure, process and outcome of care [1], is now so well known that it will not be repeated here. It is necessary to point out, however, that while this basic description is generally applicable to describing ambulatory child care programs, there are two notable exceptions: (1) The clinical relevance of care processes is usually dependent upon the age of the child. (2) Because basically healthy children are the subjects of primary child care, traditional outcome measures such as "survival" and "restoration of function" are virtually meaningless. Thus, age-dependent measures must be devised and more appropriate outcomes must be monitored.

Description of the Review System

In applying these same basic descriptive terms to evaluating the quality of a *review system*, we have extended Donabedian's Triad beyond its original application. We call the reader's attention to the fact that the parallelism described below is attributable only to us.

Structure

A quality review system for ambulatory child care is entirely dependent upon the availability of relevant age-dependent data which need to be readily available from source documents. Practical considerations usually also require that review data be in a structured format to insure completeness, handling efficiency and systematic evaluation. Needless to say, the data must first be recorded on the clinical record before they can be of any value to the review process. What that usually means is that clinicians must be much more diligent in documenting the details of the care process and its outcomes than is typically found. Review personnel, like care personnel, must be properly trained to process the data and to perform related tasks competently. Since the entire process of evaluation presumes the existence of *values*, there must also be a set of clinical goals or standards as the basis for judging the medical necessity and the clinical appropriateness of care. Typically, this calls for a set of explicit care criteria against which the record of actual care is objectively compared. Characteristic of prescriptive primary care for children, both the care process and the review process are inseparably tied to the most basic of all structural components: explicit case management objectives [2, 3].

Process

Without a built-in mechanism for actively improving the quality of source data, the prognosis for an effective review process is not very favorable. Having good data to work with requires rigorous quality control in the recording, collecting, processing and interpretation of clinical facts. This in turn calls for the mandatory correction of data errors and omissions which is preferably invoked during the process of care delivery rather than later. There must also be fixed responsibilities for correcting care deficiencies once detected, plus the careful documentation that such corrections have, in fact, been implemented. Finally, the more immediately such corrections can be invoked, the greater likelihood they will be effective in improving care.

Outcome

Contrary to common practices (especially in PSRO and related review operations [4, 5]), the direct outcome of a quality review system cannot be measured in terms of reduced hospital admissions per thousand eligibles, shortened lengths of stay, or even in increased patient survival rates. This is not because these factors necessarily relate to hospitalizations, but rather because these are all outcomes of the *care system* and not of the review system. The direct outcomes of a *review system* are more properly measured in terms of its impact on both the structure and the process by which care is delivered. Our generic term for this kind of impact is the "instrumental effectiveness" of a review system in contradistinction to its indirect impact upon patient outcomes which we would term its "ultimate effectiveness."

Thus, we would look for the direct outcomes of a quality review system to be manifested in such things as an enhanced quality of clinical data with which care providers can better assess and treat the patient (and that reviewers can also use to better assess the care that was given). A quality review system would also be sensitive in detecting deficiencies in care, effective in eliciting responsible peer judgments and capable of implementing appropriate corrective actions. It would then confirm that whatever changes were found necessary in the structure or process of the care system have, in fact, been implemented. Finally, there would be a full accountability for the review system itself in terms of its accomplishments and costs just as is expected of the care system [6].

Total Data Requirements

The total informational requirements that a comprehensive data system must meet for an ambulatory care program are dictated by four distinct and separate though interrelated functions which are (1) case management, (2) program management, (3) case evaluation and (4) program evaluation.

Case Management

This consists of all the usual clinical activities that are directly involved in caring for patients. Thus, the chief focus of data gathering is the patient and his medical characteristics. This includes not only his personal demographic profile but also important to the proper care of children is the family demographic profile and living arrangements.

The clinical data needed to properly care for well children differ considerably from the types of data needed to manage the sick child. For health maintenance activities in well children growth and development, nutrition, socialization, school performance, the current immunization status and a general physical evaluation are among the most useful data items.

In contrast to this, among sick children the classic history of the present illness, a problem-focused physical examination and a problem-specific battery of diagnostic tests are indicated.

Program Management

There is likewise a contrast in the kinds of data that are needed to manage the care program through which individual patients receive services. There are all kinds of administrative tasks involved which must be documented, such as appointment schedules, patient flow and record flow, personnel assignments and a variety of fiscal matters to be handled. In addition, the ambulatory setting in teaching hospitals also must carry out educational programs and may be, as is our own, actively engaged in a health services research program. Both these conjunctive programs carry data requirements of their own.

At this point, the foundation has been established to cite by further contrasts how the data base needed to *manage* patients differs from the kinds of data needed to *evaluate* that care.

Case Evaluation

The informational requirements for case evaluation can be summarily described as being aimed at answering questions regarding how much is known about the patient, exactly what services were provided and whether the care given was appropriate for the child's age. Thus, one needs to determine not only if a medical history was obtained, but also whether this was a complete history and one that was clinically relevant. Similar observations are needed regarding the completeness and relevancy of the physical examination and screening or laboratory tests. Because the topic under discussion deals with primary care in children, it is necessary also to determine whether the immunizations are up to date, whether the child is developing normally and whether the child-rearing practices to which he or she is exposed are appropriate for that particular child.

Once all the assessments have been completed that are appropriate to the maintenance of health in a child of a given age, then four final questions remain to be answered.

1. Are the child's health status and human potential what they should be?
2. If not, what should be done about it?
3. Were all clinically indicated interventions carried out?
4. Is there an appropraite plan for follow-up care?

In quality *assurance* programs that are worthy of the name, the evaluation activities that are designed to answer questions such as these should take place concurrently with the care process so that any care deficiencies that might be detected can be corrected while the patient is still available and the opportunity exists to improve his/her care. In all instances where the review process actively intervenes in the care process, there is a single yardstick by which it can be judged whether this intervention was appropriate. That measure is a determination of the extent to which the revised care conforms to quality standards. This is where explicit management goals (i.e., a set of age-specific care criteria) enter the picture and serve as the single standard against which the quality of care is compared and the achievements of the review system are assessed.

Program Evaluation

Just as explicit goals must be set in order to judge by comparison whether the care provided is appropriate for the individual patient, explicit goals or targets must be established for assessing the appropriateness of care provided to a given patient population whether the care setting be a hospital outpatient clinic or a practitioner's office.

The same general principles are involved in evaluating clinical care programs regardless of the setting, but the specifics of what makes an ambulatory care program good, bad or mediocre must reflect the uniqueness of both its setting and its basic care mission. Thus, the *content* of program evaluation would differ considerably when assessing the quality of primary child care in the ambulatory setting in contrast to assessing the quality of tertiary care in the hospital setting.

Evaluating the Quality of a Review System

In translating the above principles of program evaluation to monitoring the quality of a *review system* designed for use in the ambulatory care setting, a comprehensive evaluation would require adequate descriptions of its structure, process and outcomes just as it examines these aspects of a care system.

Structure

It has already been suggested that without considerable improvement in existing ambulatory care records, any serious evaluation of this care modality is virtually impossible. Thus, one of the prime structural components to be looked for in a good review system would be not only a capability for assessing the quality of source data but also the existence of some built-in mechanism to *actively improve* clinical records. Further, data management within the review system itself should be no less complete, structured, relevant, accurate and efficient than that which is expected of the care system.

Obviously, review personnel should be no less adequately trained for their specific tasks than their clinical counterparts and their responsibilities should be just as formally structured and properly designated as are those of clinicians.

Just as there must be clearly defined goals and specified management objectives for the care system, so also must exist rational and measurable management goals for the review system. Essentially, these are explicitly stated desired changes (or impacts) in the structure and processes of the care system. In practice, these take the form of specific quantifiable targets to be achieved over a discrete period of time. These, then, constitute measurable criteria by which the success or shortcomings of the review system are to be judged.

Process

Assessing the quality of review processes, as opposed to structural elements, means examining the procedures and techniques used to employ the tools, personnel and other resources the review system has at its disposal. This consists of an examination of how data are obtained from clinical records, then verified, coded, processed and evaluated. This type of assessment should look closely to see how the review personnel interpret care criteria and then obtain the data these criteria call for. It would pay special attention to the thoroughness with which data errors are searched for and the persistence with which corrections are sought.

A key determinant of the quality of a review process may well be the extent to which it acts to fix responsibility upon the clinical staff to correct whatever deficiencies in care are discovered. Another key to success will likely prove over the next few years to be the flexibility of the review process to adapt to both evolutionary changes in the way in which medicine is practiced and changes in the focus or demands placed upon review activities.

Outcome

The direct test of the quality of a review system is the measure of its *instrumental effectiveness* which we earlier defined as its capability to induce desired changes in the structure and processes of the care delivery system. In the ambulatory care setting, this would include quantifying a variety of improvements in care delivery (i.e., corrective actions) that were specifically initiated or implemented through the review process and its recommendations.

1. Enhanced quality and completeness of the outpatient record. No longer should this aspect of the patient's total care receive only cursory and unstructured documentation. Nor should the impact of ambulatory care on the patient and his family be ignored as far as recording it in the medical record is concerned.

2. Review systems that detect and report only rare or inconsequential deficiencies in care must be considered suspect. Physicians and others in the care system are human, and human oversight particularly in a busy ambulatory practice is not all that rare. A quality review system would identify all deficiencies worthy of correction within the human ability to do so. It would also do more than this.

3. It would seek out and obtain responsible peer judgments as to the nature and severity of care deficiencies and would set into motion effective means of correcting them.

4. A quality review system would not leave the implementation of recommended actions to chance but, rather, would be instrumental in bringing about needed changes.

5. Once the corrective actions have been taken, a quality review system would return to the medical record to seek confirmatory evidence that the improvements (i.e., desired changes) in the structure and the process of care delivery have, in fact, taken place.

6. A quality review system would hold itself just as accountable as the care system. It would constantly reassess its mission and reason for existence. It would also reassess the criteria by which its own success is judged. Consequently, it would periodically examine its own structure and processes and constantly strive for optimal effectiveness and maximal efficiency.

7. Finally, its ultimate responsibility is to have a positive impact upon the outcome of care. It must be recognized that review personnel are no less bound by the Hippocratic imperative "to do no harm" than are clinicians. This, too, is much too important to be left to chance and its unequivocal demonstration is perhaps the hallmark of a quality review system.

Conclusion

This paper presents a conceptual model for assessing the quality of review systems in general and focuses on those intended for use in the ambulatory setting in particular. Patterned after Donabedian's Triad, this model examines the structure, process and expected outcomes of such a review system. Data requirements for assessing the quality of primary child care were described by contrasting them with the kinds of data generated in the act of providing that care. Finally, some criteria were offered for judging the quality of a review system designed for the ambulatory setting.

References

1. Donabedian, A.: Evaluating the quality of medical care. Milbank Mem. Fund Q. 44:166-206, 1966.
2. American Academy of Pediatrics: Standards of Child Health Care, ed. 3. Evanston, Ill., 1977.

3. Frankenburg, V. and Camp, B.: Pediatric Screening Tests. Springfield, Ill.:Charles C Thomas Co., 1975.
4. Office of Professional Standards Review, U.S. Dept. of Health Education and Welfare: PSRO Program Manual, Washington, D.C., 1974, U.S. Government Printing Office.
5. Goran, M.D., Roberts, J.S., Kellogg, M.A. et al: The PSRO hospitals review system. Med. Care 13 (suppl. 4):15-75, 1975.
6. Black, G.C. and Ertel, P.Y.: Organizational issues in systematic peer review. *In* Ertel, P.Y. and Aldridge, M.G. (eds.): Medical Peer Review. St. Louis:C. V. Mosby Co., 1977, pp. 147-196.

Quality Review in Long Term Care As Conducted in North Carolina

M. Frank Sohmer, Jr., M.D. and Jean G. Barker

The purpose of this paper is to discuss the assessment of quality review in Long Term Care (LTC). The North Carolina Medical Peer Review Foundation (the Foundation) has been performing LTC review on a statewide basis for Medicaid patients since May 1973. The Foundation monitors the quality and utilization of medical services delivered under the State Plan for Medical Assistance (Title XIX) to assure that health care services are appropriate to the needs of the patients being served, are of acceptable quality and are delivered in a timely and efficient manner.

Long Term Care Review Services holds the responsibility for quality and level of care review for all Title XIX patients in mental health institutions, skilled nursing facilities, intermediate care facilities and specialty hospitals which include tuberculosis and chronic lung disease hospitals. In order to fulfill these responsibilities, a long term care review program has been developed and implemented on a statewide basis.

This review program consists of four major review mechanisms: prior approval, continued care, utilization and on-site medical review. The Foundation endorses the concept that patients should be at the appropriate level of care to promote the optimum level of rehabilitation and functioning and to serve as a cost-containment factor to the spiraling cost of health care delivery.

M. Frank Sohmer, Jr., M.D. and Jean G. Barker, North Carolina Peer Review Foundation, Raleigh.

Acknowledgments: Deana H. Beeson and Faye Castor.

Prior Approval

Prior approval is the review performed prior to entry into either a skilled nursing facility or intermediate care facility at the time of financial application for Medicaid. The purpose of prior approval is to insure that all alternative services have been considered. All Medicaid patients must be prior approved for the appropriate level of care before reimbursement can be made for services in long term care facilities.

A data abstract is utilized in completing a prior approval review. The abstract is completed to include patient information such as name, sex, Medicaid number, diagnoses, care factors and medications. The attending physician recommends a level of care and signs the request. The abstract is forwarded to the Foundation for a review by professional nurses.

Additional information is acquired by telephone contact from hospital staff, social worker or physicians as deemed appropriate. The level requested may be approved, denied or another level of care recommended following consultation with the Foundation's physician consultant and the attending physician. Following the review and assigning a prior approval number which is used for patient identification, one copy of the five page abstract is retained by the Foundation and four copies are forwarded to the county Department of Social Services. The county maintains one copy for their files and three copies are forwarded to the admitting facility. The facility completes the data processor copy and returns it to the Foundation for computer entry and reimbursement and verification.

Approximately 1,200 prior approval requests are reviewed each month with a total of 13,309 reviews conducted in 1977. The review staff will change approximately 13% of cases per month to a lower level of care. We recognize that it is very financially economical and medically beneficial to conduct a thorough review of medical care needs of a patient prior to admission to a long term care facility. Alternative services must be explored and considered before moving a person from the home environment.

In order to expedite placement, approximately 65% of the prior approval requests are completed through the telephone approval network at the Foundation.

Another service available to expedite patient placement is the *Central Bed Registry* of vacant group care beds in North Carolina. Each week an inquiry is made to each skilled nursing and intermediate care provider to determine vacant beds. The vacancy information is maintained in the Long Term Care Unit and may be requested by phone. This information is utilized by hospitals, county department of social services and physicians' offices.

An additional service provided is that of a compendium of health resources available in North Carolina, referred to as the *Community Resource Listing*. This listing provides a breakdown of resources by each of the 100 counties in North Carolina. It lists not only each specific county, but identifies the adjoining counties so that all resources nearby can be assessed. It is designed for quick, easy access for those attempting to develop discharge, transfer or admission plans for patients anywhere in North Carolina.

Continued Care Review/Utilization Review

Continued stay review is performed in conjunction with the utilization review. This is a periodic review and evaluation of the continued stay of each eligible individual receiving skilled nursing or intermediate care.

The data abstract is completed by facility nursing staff and is used as a work sheet for presenting the care needs of the patient to the Utilization Review Committee. The Committee, composed of two or more physicians, then determines the level of care required by the patient. The Foundation is responsible for monitoring the activities of the Utilization Review Committee.

There are approximately 3,000 patients reviewed per month by the Utilization Review Committees. Lower level of care changes are approximately 95 patients per month. A total of 37,874 reviews were conducted by Utilization Review Committees in 1977.

Medical Review

The purpose and function of periodic medical review is to ascertain and document whether medical assistance patients in

Title XIX skilled nursing homes, intermediate care facilities, mental hospitals and specialty hospitals are, in fact, receiving physician, skilled nursing, personal and social services for which they are eligible. The review is conducted at least annually. These services should be optimum in quality, adequate in quantity, sufficient in scope and provided in a timely manner under circumstances most favorable to the promotion of the physical, emotional, social and functional well-being of such patients.

In order to accomplish the goals as outlined for on-site medical review, North Carolina has developed and implemented a program which considers all aspects including geographical location, size, physician, and client population, number and types of facilities. Based upon this information, the concept of central office administration with geographic field teams was designed.

The central office staff provides central support and coordination of the review program. Primary responsibilities are scheduling site visits, monitoring central files, personnel administration, financial accounting and correspondence with the state, facilities and review teams.

Each review team is composed of a registered nurse, medical social worker and a physician. There are presently seven teams in four geographic locations. The physician consultant is a practicing physician from the geographical area of the facility being reviewed. The physician has prime responsibility for performance of the team and for medical evaluation and all recommendations resulting from a review. The registered nurse makes determinations regarding quality and appropriateness of nursing care rendered. The medical social worker is trained in the social factors of illness and evaluates the social and psychological needs of each patient.

Each on-site review is scheduled 60 days in advance. The facility is notified no more than 48 hours in advance and in the event of a follow-up review, no notice may be given.

The following outlines the sequence of events of an on-site review:

The entrance interview is conducted for the purpose of introducing team members to key facility staff, explaining the purpose and procedures to be followed and identifying sources of information available in the facility.

Each patient will be assessed regarding his medical, nursing, social, psychological and functioning level.

The medical social worker reviews the patient's records including social histories, social progress notes, social plan of care and activity program assessment. All social and psychological aspects of the patient are considered.

The nurse reviews the entire chart of each patient including all records used in patient care such as the cardex. Documentation is reviewed for compliance as required by federal regulations. However, the review team is interested to see not only that the patient has a history, physical and discharge summary, but that they give pertinent and complete data concerning the patient. Likewise, the chart is reviewed for physician orders, progress notes, laboratory work and notes by other disciplines as well as the patient care plan.

After reviewing the charts of all patients, the team has an overall view of the medical/social supervision, how the disciplines work together and whether pertinent information concerning the patient is documented, such as laboratory work and physical therapy.

The nurse and medical social worker then visit each patient with a facility staff member.

A summary of the observations and facts collected on each patient is then dictated by the nurse and medical social worker.

After the nurse and medical social worker have visited all patients, a conference is held. At this time, they discuss any patient on which they may have a question concerning his care. A possible recommendation is formulated and a referral form is initiated on each patient, which is to be seen by the physician consultant.

The physician consultant visits on the last day of the review. The nurse and the medical social worker relate to him an overview of what they have found during the entire review concerning the medical supervision, nursing care in general and social aspects of care in the facility.

The patients that have been selected for the physician to visit are reviewed with the possible recommendations by the nurse and the social worker. The physician consultant will also review a sampling of charts for which no possible recommendation has been formulated. The entire team then visits these selected patients and a conference is held. The physician then makes his recommendations. He always makes the final decision and recommendation.

After the team has completed the visits, an exit conference is held with the team members, the administrator, nursing director, social service designee and/or activities director and anyone else who might benefit from this. At this time, a complete verbal report is given, which includes everything that will be included in the final written report, which will be mailed out in approximately five days following the review. The report is sent to the administrator, the utilization review chairman, the consulting physician and the state regulatory agencies.

There are four types of recommendations which may result from an on-site medical review. These are as follows:

1. General recommendations are those to improve the quality of care for the total patient population.

2. Problem areas are those which enumerate state and federal laws/regulations not being complied with.

3. Patient recommendations are specific to the needs of a particular patient.

4. Level of care recommendations indicate if the patient's needs are being met at the current level of care, or if the patient should be at an alternate level of care.

On-site review statistics for 1977 are as follows:

- 14,232 patients reviewed
- 1,334 patient recommendations
- 1,950 facility recommendations
- 549 change in level of care recommendations

At present, North Carolina has approximately 19,000 Title XIX certified beds in 280 facilities.

Physician

The North Carolina Medical Peer Review Foundation is a physician-founded and physician-oriented organization dedicated to the concept of peer review for all services and for all disciplines of care.

Membership is open to any physician licensed to practice in North Carolina and now totals over 2,000. The Foundation is governed by a board of directors composed of 18 practicing physicians who oversee the administrative actions of the organization.

The Committee on Norms of Care is composed of 15 physicians representing the major speciality fields. In addition, the Committee is assisted by 19 subspecialty advisors. The Committee is responsible for making decisions on medical policy, patterns of care and individual questions on utilization review. The Committee meets regularly to develop medical policy, establish standards of care, conduct peer review and provide appellant review.

The Subcommittee on Nursing Home Criteria is composed of four members from the Committee on Norms of Care. These physicians have practicing experience in the areas of the elderly, long term disabled and the service system available for these persons. Their responsibilities include development of criteria for long term care patients, providing an appellant mechanism for attending physicians and patient/families in LTC review, developing policies, providing periodic reports to the Committee on Norms of Care and serving as physician liaison for the Foundation in the long term care setting.

In the Long Term Care Review Program, approximately 100 different consultants are utilized involving 900 hours of physician time. Physician guidance and participation in each type of review is as follows:

1. In the areas of Prior Approval, Continued Care Review, and Utilization Review, the Foundation has available an inhouse consultant. This physician is responsible for the review of any problem case, at which time he will discuss the patient's care needs with the attending physician and utilization review committee as appropriate, in order to render an objective level of care recommendation. He also serves as the first level of appellant review in those cases where the Utilization Review Committee and physician cannot agree and in those cases where an attending physician disagrees with the reviewing staff regarding a prior authorization or continued stay review.

2. A physician consultant is utilized in each on-site medical review. In this role, he serves as the review team's director, programmer and coordinator and is the final authority for its medical finding, patient-care recommendations and official actions. His special function is to review and assess the physician services and the medical management of each patient's case by attending physicians. The physician consultant contacts attending physicians, at the time of the review, to

discuss the team's observations and recommendations pertinent to their patients. He also serves as the first level of appellant review, should an attending physician disagree with level of care recommendations. His general responsibility is the supervision of the review team's visit to assure that observations are sufficient to make the necessary judgments regarding the quality of care for each patient.

With the tremendous support and active participation of the physicians in North Carolina, the Foundation believes that peer review has become available in its truest form and has indeed improved the quality of life for North Carolina citizens while being cost-effective. Foundation physician consultants have also provided in-service and continuing education on specific topics for facilities such as foot care, decubitus care, oral hygiene and urological care.

Future of Long Term Care Review

The two greatest factors affecting the future of LTC review will be federal regulation and funding. Current regulations discourage cost-effective review mechanisms. Quality and cost-effective review could be accomplished if some provisions were made for judgment to reduce review frequency and review composition in facilities known to be providing outstanding care.

Federal regulations mandate that conditionally designated PSROs assume responsibility for LTC review within two years of designation. Funding LTC review for PSROs has been haphazard at best. Our experience has been that quality review mechanisms are implemented but that the data collection mechanism and reporting systems more often fail to materialize due to funding rstrictions and regulation changes. The waste that results is inexcusable.

Any review system that services over the next ten years must include documentation of cost effectiveness. Our long term care review program in the fiscal year 1978 cost the state of North Carolina $713,000 and documented a cost savings of $3,764,000.

All in all, the future for long term care review has more unknowns than knowns. We feel confident that some type of review will continue. The structure will be dependent upon the legislative process and appropriations.

Measures and Analyses for an Experimental Evaluation of Quality Assurance Mechanisms

David B. Maglott, M.H.A., Linda V. Esrov, Ph.D.,
Robert W. Hetherington, Ph.D. and
Phyllis J. Pallett, M.P.H.

The Division of Intramural Research, National Center for Health Services Research (NCHSR), in collaboration with the Division of Hospitals and Clinics, Bureau of Medical Services, is conducting a study to evaluate the effectiveness of peer review mechanisms intended to assess and assure the quality of hospital care. Although extensive developmental and demonstration efforts have been directed toward various protocols for peer review, there is as yet no convincing evidence for their efficacy in improving the quality of medical care in hospitals. The present study was designed to determine whether several recently developed protocols for peer review, using explicit criteria for the quality of care, can be shown to be more effective than a control protocol designed to be as comprehensive as possible without the use of explicit quality of care criteria.

The peer review mechanisms chosen for evaluation include (a) a retrospective review model similar to the medical care evaluation studies required by JCAH and PSRO, (b) a concurrent review model generally thought to have potential for altering physician behavior and (c) the combination of these two. All three of these mechanisms employ condition-specific explicit criteria for the quality of care which are used as

David B. Maglott, M.H.A., Linda V. Esrov, Ph.D., Robert W. Hetherington, Ph.D. and Phyllis J. Pallett, M.P.H., Evaluation of Alternative Review Systems (EARS) Project, Division of Intramural Research, National Center for Health Services Research, Hyattsville, Md.

guidelines by nonphysician personnel to select those cases that are at variance with the criteria so that they can be reviewed by physicians. While the physician review component of the mechanisms is not significantly different from more traditional systems, the use of the criteria and the nonphysician personnel to screen cases represents significant innovations. The control mechanism includes physician review of cases concurrently and retrospectively, but without the use of either explicit criteria or the ancillary personnel to screen cases for review.

The additions of explicit medical care criteria and nonphysician personnel to physician peer review techniques, and the simultaneous formalization of the traditionally informal organization of the physician review process, have greatly increased the costs of doing peer review. These increased costs include both the obvious costs of criteria development, extra personnel, data systems and administrative structures, and the less obvious but very real opportunity costs involved in diverting nursing, medical record, data management and administrative personnel to this quality assurance function. If it can be demonstrated that these new mechanisms are significantly more effective in improving the practice of medicine than a more traditional peer review approach, the added costs may be justified. Further, if it can be shown in which specific areas the various review mechanisms are effective, intelligent choices could be made about the most effective and efficient ways of assuring adequate levels of quality of care.

Each of the four peer review mechanisms will be used in two hospitals of the U.S. Public Health Service, as shown in Table 1.

The criteria to be employed in the explicit review models are based in part on previous research and development funded by NCHSR, such as the Experimental Medical Care Review Organization (EMCRO) program. After reviewing that work, the research team suggested a criteria structure which seemed to be both useful as a conceptual framework and reflective of the various issues to be raised in reviewing care. With minor changes, representatives of the six test hospitals accepted this format, which covers the justification for admission; validation of the diagnosis; justification for specified surgeries and special procedures; critical elements of history, physical exam, diag-

Table 1. Treatment and Control Groups for Evaluation of Alternative Review Systems

Study Group		*Peer Review Mechanism*
Treatment #1	(2 Hospitals)	Concurrent and retrospective quality assurance review mechanisms
Treatment #2	(2 Hospitals)	Concurrent quality assurance review mechanisms only
Treatment #3	(2 Hospitals)	Retrospective quality assurance review mechanisms only
Control	(2 Hospitals)	Structured, implicit quality assurance review mechanisms

nostic tests and procedures, and therapy; other noncritical elements in those categories; contraindicated diagnostic and therapeutic elements; the prevention of complications; the occurrence and treatment of complications; length of stay; and discharge status of the patient. The physician investigators from the test hospitals, with data and help from the interagency research team, then identified 25 potential conditions for review. Factors used in selecting these conditions included their frequencies of occurrence across the hospitals, the precision with which they could be defined, the availability of a definable and effective regimen of therapy and potential morbidity or mortality of the condition. The selections also included a conscious effort to balance conditions across the major departments. The criteria for these conditions have been developed by the staffs of the six test hospitals, starting within each staff and later being resolved at meetings of representatives of each of six staffs.

The explicit medical care review mechanisms which act as treatments in this design are also the products of earlier research and development funded by NCHSR. Under the EMCRO program, prototype retrospective and concurrent review models of inpatient quality assurance mechanisms were developed and tested in multiple settings. This current research project attempts to pull together the best features of those models to form optimal prototypes for testing, both individually and in combination. All three models focus only on assessing and assuring the quality of medical care, with particular emphasis on analyzing variations to determine whether they are justifiable because of patient characteristics or whether they indicate deficiencies. Quality Assurance Committees have been established by each of the Medical Staffs to coordinate the respective review processes, to supervise the analysis of problems and to suggest and monitor corrective measures.

The retrospective review model involves periodic and frequent condition-specific audits, at the rate of about one a month per hospital. The audits are divided across the major departments of medicine and surgery and are conducted on a departmental basis. Data are abstracted by medical record personnel from recently discharged cases. These data are presented to the department, with specific attention to cases in which the process of care is at variance with the criteria developed to screen cases with that admission diagnosis. The departmental staff then analyzes the data, determining for each such variation whether some characteristics of the patient and his problem indicate the variation is a justifiable exception to the criteria or whether the variation indicates a deficiency in the process of care. For all deficiencies, the staff then determines to whom or to what set of factors to assign responsibility and estimates the most likely cause of the deficiency. Based on this analysis and considering any patterns of problems which emerge, the staff recommends to the Quality Assurance Committee the necessary actions to correct the problems it has identified. After a reasonable period of attempting to correct the problems, new data on the process of care, collected as before, are presented to the staff. Using the same process, the staff again determines whether problems exist and, specifically, whether previously targeted problems have been corrected. The process is repeated until the process of care is acceptable to the staff.

The concurrent review process employs trained nurse reviewers to screen cases during treatment. Whenever an apparent variation from the screening criteria occurs, the nurse, after seeking any necessary clarification from the attending physician, refers the matter to one of several physician advisers. The physician adviser reviews the chart, may discuss the matter with the attending physician and determines whether the variation, if confirmed, is a justifiable exception because of unique characteristics of the patient and his problems. If the variation is not justified, the deficiency in the process of care is reviewed with the attending physician to determine what can be done to correct it and to assure that all necessary actions are taken. An appeals mechanism is available to the attending physician. The physician adviser will periodically report both his decisions on variations and his attempts to correct deficiencies to the Quality Assurance Committee, which will review the deficiencies noted to determine whether additional efforts are needed to prevent their future recurrence.

The combined review mechanism, employing both retrospective and concurrent review, uses both mechanisms to identify problems in care that need correction and integrates the findings in the Quality Assurance Committee. The Committee can then use both of the mechanisms to monitor the efficacy of its attempt to correct problems.

The control treatment involves physician review of a sample of inpatient charts on the third day after admission and post-discharge review of an overlapping sample of cases. No prephysician screening of cases is used, and no explicit review criteria are employed. The reviewing physician looks at all aspects of care to determine whether, in his judgment, there are areas where the process of care should have been better. For currently active cases, these areas, together with any other questionable aspects of the case, are discussed by the reviewing and attending physicians. The results, and the results of the review of discharged cases, are presented to the Quality Assurance Committee, which must decide what additional problem areas or patterns of problems need correcting.

The major question being addressed in this study is the relative amount of change in physician behavior that is achieved in each of these review models. The hypothesis behind the new explicit criteria-based models is that they bring about greater change in physician behavior than the more traditional implicit approach. To examine this, we propose to use an unweighted measure of compliance to criteria for quality of care as a measure of explicit behavioral change. Because the explicit models review care on a diagnosis-specific basis using the principal diagnosis as the mechanism for classification, the initial comparisons will be condition-specific and then will be segmented within and across conditions for similar aspects of care, e.g., justification of admission, prevention and treatment of complications. Medical and surgical cases will be examined separately for differences in effect of review. It would also be useful to compare the changes in behavior achieved in reviewed conditions with any change in behavior which may occur simultaneously in nonreviewed cases.

The implicit model reviews a sample of cases across all diagnoses on the assumption that the types of problems found in the sample are representative of those in the other cases and on the assumption that alterations in behavior achieved in reviewed cases will carry over to nonreviewed cases. The same measure of behavioral change is proposed in this model on the assumption that the iterative process of developing criteria that was employed in the six test hospitals produced criteria that are also generally reflective of the thinking of the physicians in the control hospitals. Thus, changes in the compliance of behavior to the explicit criteria will be used to assess behavioral change here, too. Particularly important here will be condition-specific comparisons between reviewed and nonreviewed cases with the same principal diagnosis. It should be noted here that this measure of compliance to the criteria, as discussed, is specifically a measure of behavior and not of the quality of the behavior, i.e., it is not being used as a measure of the quality of the process of care.

If it can be demonstrated that peer review alters the behavior of physicians, the next question is whether these changes in the behavior of physicians are medically significant: i.e., do they improve the quality of the process of care. The question of medical significance implies some sort of weighting of the various criterion items, recognizing both that some items are of greater importance in achieving desired outcomes than others and that different types of items contribute to different objectives (e.g., items that facilitate the making of the diagnosis vs. those that are therapeutic for that diagnostic condition). There are several ways to approach this weighting problem. The most direct is to focus on those aspects of care which the reviewing physicians found to be deficient on the assumption that the decision to try to correct such deficiencies is based on the opinion that the element of care is significant in its contribution to achieving outcomes and that its absence, therefore, means the outcomes of care may be less than desired. By this approach, only change in compliance to targeted problem criteria would be considered, and this would provide a basic measure of the impact of peer review on the quality of the process of care.

Because this approach is limited to those cases determined to be deficient, and because those areas may not be the same across hospitals or across treatment groups, providing unclear comparisons, several other techniques for weighting behavior changes by significance are also being considered. These include the possibility of assigning weighted values to all criterion items on the basis of concensual agreement and the possibility of empirical derivation of weights by the relative contribution to definable short-term outcomes. The former approach might be similar to the kind used several years ago by Payne in the application of his Physician Performance Index, where weights in the 1-3 range were used, or might involve selecting only the most critical aspects of care by effectively assigning 0 or 1 values to the items. The problem with this approach is that the iterative cross-hospital process used to identify the explicit criteria in this study may already have reduced the criteria to a core of nearly equivalent items. The second approach is conceptually more attractive: combining the focused weighting (0,1) approach with a regression technique in which key process elements are related to a small number of specific short-term outcome measures in an attempt to assess empirically the relative contributions (weights of criterion items). Obviously, the difficulties involved in assessing short-term outcomes and the possibility that the process criteria items and the chosen outcome measures are not related make this approach somewhat questionable.

In addition to examining the comparative effects that different peer review models have on physician behavior and the quality of the process of care, the study also examines the effects the different models have on several measures of outcomes. As a generic measure of outcome, we are employing a function status measure modified from work by Bush and Anderson and including a modified version of the Katz ADL scale. We will be looking at the impact of review on the level of function status at and post-discharge as well as the impact of review on the amount of change in function status from admission to discharge and admission to a fixed point post-admission. One would hypothesize that a higher quality of care might lead to improved function status at discharge and at a constant time after admission, when admission status and length of stay are held constant. While there are several different patterns of change in function status that would be expected for different disease types, it is not clear that all of these patterns are truly effected by the medical care process. Certainly for some conditions, therefore, changes in the quality of medical care might not demonstrate significant changes in function status.

For this reason we are also attempting to measure the impact of the various review models in terms of improvements in defined short-term outcomes specific to various conditions and diagnoses. While there are significant difficulties in defining measurable short-term outcomes, the theoretical link between changes in the process of care and changes in the outcomes of care seems to make it worth the effort.

As the final outcome measure, the study will examine whether the various peer review models can achieve patient-visible improvements in the quality of the process and outcomes of care, the hypothesis being that changes in these areas are/can be visible to the patient population, so that patient perceptions of the quality of care (patient satisfaction with care) will improve as review continues. This measure builds on work by Ware and others, which indicates that not only is patient satisfaction a multidimensional construct, but that within the quality of care dimension, patients can distinguish between the quality of the technical aspects of care and the quality of the human-art aspects of care. We are specifically attempting to measure the impact of the various peer review models in each of these latter areas.

Another variable of interest is the value of services utilized during the inpatient stay. The peer review models used in this study are designed as quality assurance mechanisms and not as cost-control mechanisms. Nevertheless, it is important to study the impact of this kind of review on the utilization of services, for there are two very different schools of thought on the likely outcome. One hypothesis is that improving the quality of care by bringing physician behavior into compliance with explicit criteria for the quality of medical care will cause the number of services to increase, thereby increasing the value of services utilized. A second broad hypothesis is that improving the quality of care by increasing compliance to criteria for good quality care decreases the total utilization of services by focusing attention on the appropriate services and increasing the efficiency of medical care in the early part of the hospital stay. In order to assess this value of services rendered, we are itemizing the services provided and weighting them by their relative values. This process will give us the weighted values of services rendered by major categories (radiology, laboratory, etc.) and frees us of the difficulties of comparing costs of services across hospitals with variable cost structures.

In addition to the various dependent variables, there are a large number of explanatory or control variables which need to be considered. Foremost among these are those describing differences in the patient populations across treatment groups, hospitals and diagnostic categories. The large proportion of American seamen and active duty military personnel seen at several of our hospitals contrasts sharply with the retired military and military-dependent personnel seen at some hospitals or the aged and medically indigent population seen at others. The racial and sex distributions also differ significantly. In specific medical aspects, preliminary analysis in one diagnosis already indicates that the admitting level function status differs significantly across hospitals. Such factors might be expected to influence the types of variations from the criteria which would be found (behavior) as well as the review decisions about whether the variations are justifiable (quality of the process of care). These factors and the presence of other condition-specific prognostic risk factors may also have a significant impact on the specific outcomes achieved, on the changes in function status which can be expected, on the patient's perception of the quality of his care and on the utilization of services.

Besides these patient population differences, some of the same factors and others must be considered in analyzing patient care even within the same diagnostic category in one hospital. A shift in the smoking habits of surgical patients, for example, might produce a change in outcomes achieved that is quite independent of the process of care delivered. Similarly, a patient with extensive co-morbid illness may require considerably more services than a patient with the same principal diagnosis who has no other health problems, regardless of the quality of the care delivered for the principal diagnosis. Similarly, a patient who is generally satisfied with life may have a very different perception of the care he has received than one who finds his life quite disappointing.

It is also important to be able to control for differences between the physicians treating different cases. Factors such as specialty, board status and number of years after training have all been shown to influence the process of care. The possibility exists that these factors may also influence the ability to alter the process of care and therefore may limit or facilitate the ability of a particular review mechanism to alter physician behavior. The association between physician characteristics and the changes produced will be watched carefully.

Finally, the characteristics of the hospitals themselves will undoubtedly influence both the operation and success of the review mechanisms. Staffing patterns, staffing shortages, specialty distributions, training programs and affiliations might all limit the degree or type of change which can be produced or maintained in any setting. In addition, several organizational variables such as internal communication, coordination and degree of specification of procedures have been shown to bear directly on the outcomes of care achieved. It will therefore be important to monitor both cross-hospital differences and changes within each hospital over time.

The design of the data collection process — and the explicit review process — is shown in Figure 1. The design started with a period of nonreview to allow stabilization of the behavior of physicians. Baseline data collection then began in February 1976 in five conditions. The data set for these conditions included patient demographic characteristics; utilization of services; a concurrent assessment of compliance to criteria at specific times; a retrospective assessment of overall compliance to the criteria requirements; and determinations of the patient's function status at admission, discharge and at six weeks after

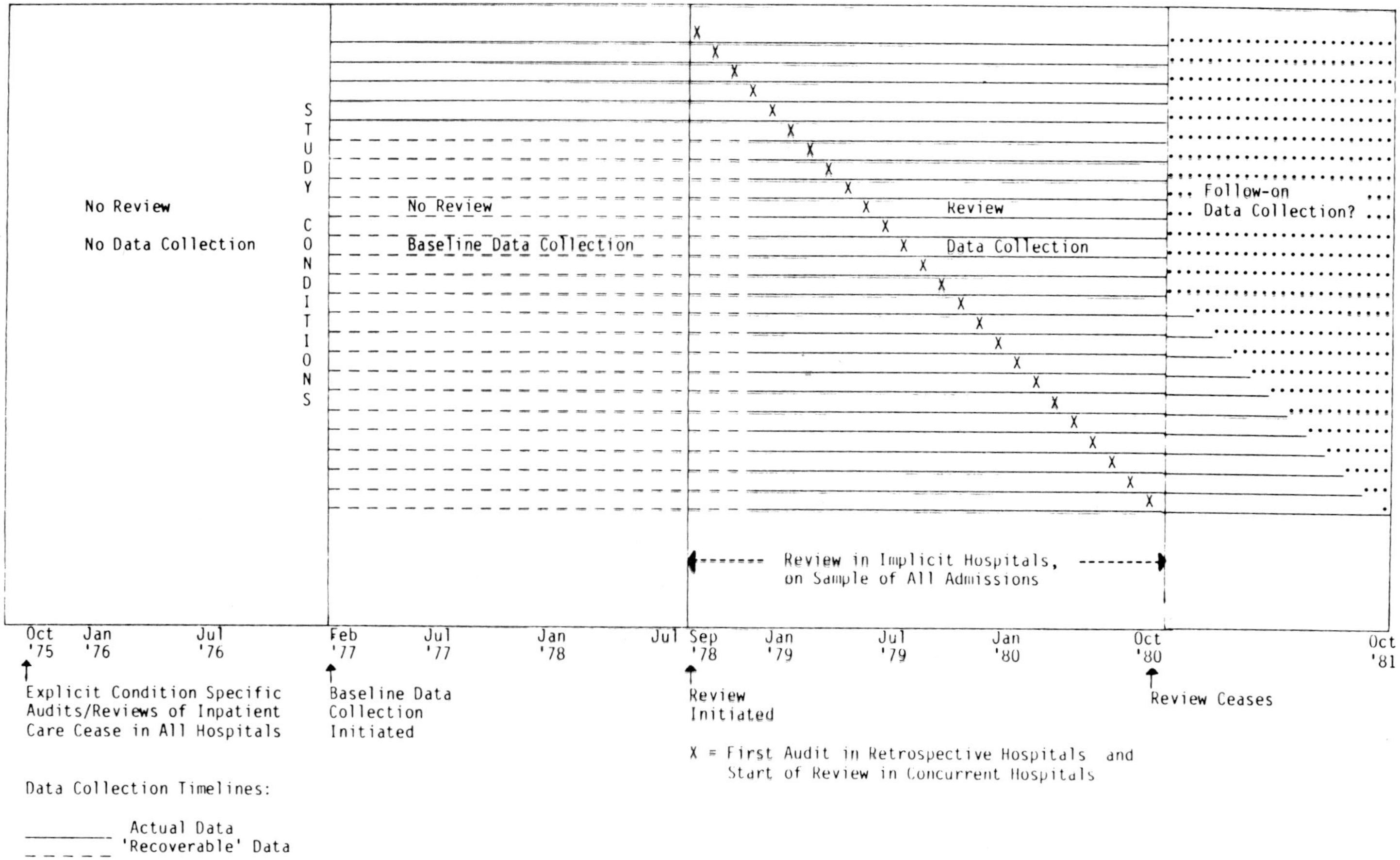

No Review

No Data Collection

STUDY CONDITIONS

No Review

Baseline Data Collection

Review

Data Collection

Follow-on
Data Collection?

Review in Implicit Hospitals,
on Sample of All Admissions

Oct '75 | Jan '76 | Jul '76 | Feb '77 | Jul '77 | Jan '78 | Jul | Sep '78 | Jan '79 | Jul '79 | Jan '80 | Oct '80 | Oct '81

Explicit Condition Specific
Audits/Reviews of Inpatient
Care Cease in All Hospitals

Baseline Data
Collection
Initiated

Review
Initiated

Review Ceases

X = First Audit in Retrospective Hospitals and
Start of Review in Concurrent Hospitals

Data Collection Timelines:

——— Actual Data
– – – 'Recoverable' Data

FIG. 1. Data collection and medical care review design in the Evaluation of Alternative Review Systems (EARS) Project.

admission. Data on patient satisfaction and condition-specific prognostic risk and outcome factors were not collected during most of the baseline period.

The start of peer review activities occurred in September 1978. In the explicit review models, the design calls for sequential introduction of review on successive diagnoses over a two-year period, with another year of follow-up. In the implicit model, the design requires review of a sample of all cases designed to yield the same intensity of review over the two years as that achieved in the explicit hospitals.

The selection of the 25 diagnostic categories or conditions made two years ago by the physician investigators was handicapped by having to work with data on the discharge diagnoses of patients as opposed to the principal diagnosis. Unfortunately, this means that there are, in fact, not enough cases in some categories at some hospitals to allow us to use the conditions for analysis — or even, in some cases, to allow peer review to be conducted at all. However, there are enough useful conditions to allow us the intended 10 to 12 diagnoses for condition-specific analyses and a large number (18 to 20?) for cross-condition comparisons (and review).

Factors in Successful and Failed Computing Projects in Medicine

Prof. J. Anderson, D. J. Cooper and A. Nimalasurya

Introduction

An important aspect of any real endeavor is the innovative objectives with which it sets out and it is hoped will be realized over a period of time. In the research field in medicine most projects produce new data, but it is usually an amplification or a derivation of existing knowledge. This is so in the pharmaceutical industry, for example, where 90% or more of proposed new drugs are not strictly new departures. Rarely do such projects succeed in opening up totally new areas of exploration, but those that just amplify are important in adding to the stock of existing knowledge and to provide the basis from which the leaps in our knowledge occur.

So it is with medical computing. Most future projects will be derived from existing projects. Spencer [1] in his survey of medical computer projects that have been operating over the last decade or more found that most were in the area of hospital billing and administration or in the projection of statistics describing health care. The next significant developments were in the clinical laboratories where the analysis of results from automated machines was obtained and by computer signal analysis of biological signals; the electrocardiogram is an example. Fewer were those projects that were concerned with strictly limited aspects of patient care, medical records and special aspects of medical theory such as diagnostic classification, drug classification and drug side effects.

Prof. J. Anderson, D. J. Cooper and A. Nimalasurya, Department of Medicine, King's College Hospital Medical School, Denmark Hill, London, England.

Considerable experience in the application of information processing had been gained in areas outside medicine, especially in commerce and banking, before the applications in the medical field became extensive. Methods and packages transferred from these areas except in medical administration usually led to project failure, but they have highlighted the inadequacies and difficulties of medical procedures. They are useful, too, when they indicate what other alternatives may be pursued.

General Observations

In any discussion of the success and failure of medical computing projects it is essential to see why such endeavors are both necessary and useful to medicine. In recent years there has been an information explosion resulting from the application of scientific research to all aspects of medicine and related sciences. One response to this has been the reductionist approach of defining an increasing number of medical specialities and, by doing so, brought the information span within the competence of an individual physician.

A new alternative approach is for some of the data processing and memory storage functions of the physician to be taken over by computer systems and for these systems to be used to provide the information that he needs in the solution of the patients' health care problems [2].

It is not surprising that mistakes are made and that there are failures in determining the best methods. By the very nature of the inquiry not all projects will have a successful outcome, yet all will yield pertinent data even if some only show that certain approaches are not appropriate. Many aspects of projects in medical computing resemble projects in clinical research, a field that is already familiar. Many of the concepts behind the assessment of medical computing projects for support and evaluation were taken from the past procedures in medical research. Unfortunately, there are big differences in the time scales that are required for achieving significant results.

That there would be difficulties in areas in medicine concerned with information processing and involving a significant number of systems was to be expected. These problems occurred in system design, the choice of hardware and the development of appropriate software and in implementation. The problems were compounded by the fact that the time requirements were often not thoroughly understood by either the sponsors, computer manufacturers or by those undertaking the research.

There was another problem that arose because of the expense of the basic hardware and software from the computer manufacturers. It was felt that payment required was so great that it could not be justified for systems confirmed to an individual research project and that systems that were developed should be able, in a short time period, to be implemented as standard projects in the health care system. In other words, the pressure was created by the sponsors, very often governments or governmental agencies, to rush newly researched systems from the research field through the development stage to implementation as rapidly as possible and thus demonstrate a return on the investment.

It also became apparent that those who sponsored such research were taking concepts from industry into a field where basic constraints and outcomes were not the same. Indeed, in so far as drug development was concerned, industry took over from basic research in the medical science departments in medical schools and they developed the products to standard production levels. Thus, medical research workers unused to such a system were being asked not only to do research, but to operate under a whole set of new conditions.

There was an additional factor for those considering the implementation of a computer system that the computer manufacturer, unlike the makers of laboratory equipment, had to sell general purpose machines to all his customers and viewed the medical field in the same way as he considered areas such as banking, commerce and local government. Consequently the hardware needs of medical projects did not always correspond with what was available and these difficulties often caused projects to deviate from their objectives.

Additionally, the manufacturer was responsible for the basic software for the operating and filing systems (and, more recently, for the data base system) and for the design of the hardware and software for the peripheral interfaces with the users. Thus, to a large extent, the manufacturer defined the man-machine interface. It is obvious that the proper function of the hardware and basic software was vital. One of the common sources of large unforeseen costs and even project failure was repeated hardware or software malfunction.

A further problem identified is in the area of project evaluation; many sponsors of medical information projects seem to be obsessed with evaluation. They felt that the standard method of project evaluation by publication and by group review was inadequate and that the large capital expenditure required a different type of evaluation to justify the nature of the investment. Thus, project evaluation often had to be inbuilt into a project and this was a costly overhead. Elsewhere, teams were set up by sponsors, usually government Departments of Health, so they could evaluate the results of projects and attempt to protect the investment. Detailed analysis of cost-effectiveness assumed enormous importance and the saving of part of the salary of a clerk or secretary appeared to be more vital than the fact that such projects were going to change the whole concept of medicine and develop entirely new and different ways of approaching health care. Such evaluations tended to ignore the fact that the most important change was ecological.

Project Implementation

In designing the objectives for a computer project, not only have the detailed cognitive aspects to be laid bare, but the objectives have to take into account policy decisions at local and regional level and to anticipate the future use of the system which is being designed. Also to be considered are the means by which the system interfaces with physicians and nurses. It is unlikely that the objectives, procedures and methods adopted after all these factors have been taken into account will be the same as those originally conceived.

Overall, the choice of objectives is crucial to the project and often the care with which such statements are constructed decides its ultimate success or failure. Because of the relatively high cost of medical computing research, there is the tendency for sponsors to want objectives designed to meet their requirements rather than those of the people who are about to undertake the research. There is also the problem of understanding technical language; in some projects objectives have had to be reduced from explicit statements to more implicit statements and to a level where lay sponsors can have some general ideas about the project. Usually this means that the objectives lose specificity, something that is so important for the appropriate design of software [3].

Different hardware and software solutions are not commonly entertained or investigated. Indeed, in some projects it is obvious that issues about objectives have been decided by the types of hardware and software that have been available. At this early stage the user interface of the new system usually receives little attention and the tendency to ignore the human context of medical information systems has been one of the important causes of project failure.

Resources

The matching of objectives to the required resources of hardware, software, systems and programming teams is one that is difficult to achieve successfully, especially if the project is in one of the more difficult and poorly explored areas of medical information systems. There is a tendency on the part of sponsors to assume that by pouring in more human resources the work is completed more quickly and cheaply. Generally this is not true; projects have to be managed and the greater the management task the less time will be available for the leader to devote to achieving the research objectives.

It has to be borne in mind when choosing the resources that the required balance might vary through the duration of the project. Some people are good at research and pushing systems forward and others are more suited to development and implementation of such projects. Therefore, it is important that the human resources be matched to the progression of the objectives as they unfold in the course of the project. Errors here can create considerable human conflict and this tends to bring the project into jeopardy. There is a tendency for sponsors to push leaders into situations that are not appropriate to their talents and are surprised when resources are not applied or managed correctly. Additionally, it is often not appreciated by sponsors that lay committees are not the proper way either to guide and organize research. Research needs leaders and not balanced, time-wasting committees. There are many pitfalls in relation to resources and their correct utilization. Correctly used resources make the pathway to success easier; when mismanaged the tendency toward project failure increases.

Systems Implementation

This is an important area from the point of view of organizing appropriate implementation, controlling the research and development and also of matching hardware and software requirements with the tasks to be implemented. The other side of the problem, often ignored or played down by those responsible for the implementation, is the necessity for obtaining the cooperation and confidence of the users. This can be done only if there is an appropriate understanding and commitment on both sides.

The users are expected to change their ways of working, often fairly radically, to meet the requirements of the new man-machine interface. This has usually been a teletypewriter or a keyboard which leads to a visual display unit or other device to display information. The systems for accepting information are often rather restricted and lack flexibility. Most offer a "menu selection" type of choice or response to questionnaires (usually of the yes — no variety) or text with blank spaces to be filled in. Flexible methods of data entry are not usually allowed because of software limitations. Naturally, the user expects a return for the extra effort required.

The output to be returned to the user has always been a difficult problem in medical records, since textual reports are required from the bulk of the entered data. The users are being asked to be more accurate and more specific but in return are usually offered only simple tabulations of data and may receive little encouragement to compensate for their extra efforts. This has proved to be one of the most intractable problems, but where appropriate it may be possible to compensate some users by, for example, the timely return of investigative results.

Naturally, user education is essential especially in a hospital, and this needs to be an ongoing process. As projects grow and develop so the users' acceptance of and ideas about the system increase. What was once acceptable to the user later becomes drudgery. This can be changed only by education and motivation — something requiring dedicated effort and time. Unfortunately, users and most sponsors underrate resources that are needed to be committed to this task. Often the success or failure of projects is decided by the way the users are motivated.

Evaluation

This is a problem for project sponsors. Lay committees have been selected for this purpose but either they only serve to do the wishes of the project team or they tend to interfere with project leadership and submit the project to intolerable strains. The changing by the committee of the objectives of a project without consulting the sponsors is not unknown and this inevitably leads to project failure at a later date. The selection of an appropriate evaluation system is costly because it is necessary to create a team sufficiently competent to understand and cope with the project. Groups of consultants are, on the whole, too involved elsewhere to function as members of such a team for any length of time although individual consultants may be successfully included.

More often than not, investigation of whether the objectives and time scales are being met should be a continuing monitoring process rather than set evaluations at fixed intervals. It should be noted that very often original estimates of time scales are highly optimistic and the problems that are likely to occur in implementation are often grossly underestimated.

The past conflicts about batch and interactive processing are now behind us. The emphasis is now on using the best techniques to solve the task in hand; nevertheless, preconceived ideas in evaluation teams can lead to problems for project leaders and create dissatisfaction on both sides. Such dissension tends to slow projects down and provides a focus for deviation from the objectives and consequent failure.

Management

The management of research projects has always been a problem. Most active research workers do not want to get involved in development and implementation of their research but would rather go on to test new ideas. Thus, the project leadership has to resolve this problem since people are necessary for implementation as well as for research. This calls for firm leadership and also a well-defined set of objectives agreed to by all.

It is important that these objectives are universally understood and accepted. Repeated reporting to numerous committees and continual reinterpretation and changing of objectives by higher management can only lead to chaos. Support from the sponsor should be consistent to sustain the leadership until the project is completed. Many mistakes have been made in projects because of failure of the sponsors to do this. Proper project management is essential and failure here is likely to mean failure to the project.

Ecology

Hospitals are active institutions with system and direction established by tradition. Institutions are slow to change; if medical information systems are to be a success, a large number of people in the institution must cooperate in the development of the systems and be aware of its advantages and usefulness. There is a need for a general education in the institution as well as the specific education of users. These are important aspects of success. To provide encouragement to all those in the institution who have an interest in the project a public relations exercise is needed and common courtesy calls for the project's progress and results to be conveyed to these people.

Conclusion

Overall success or failure in large information system projects is not determined by one particular difficulty. Usually there is a multitude of problems occurring in many of the areas outlined, and mistakes in one area may be propagated to several others. Research we must have and learn from our failures.

References

1. Spencer, W.A.: An opinion survey of computer applications in 149 hospitals in U.S.A., Europe and Japan. Med. Inform. 1976, pp. 215-234.
2. Collen, M.F.: General Requirements and Accepted Computer Systems. New York:J. Wiley & Sons, 1976, pp. 3-23.
3. Wasserman, A.I.: A problem-list of public policy aims concerning computers and health care. Comm. ACM 18:279-280, 1975.

Acute-Care Psychiatric Beds Needs Assessment

Jack LaPatra, Ph.D.

The Impact of Certificate of Need

The literature listed [1-14] evolved for two major reasons. First, mental health needs assessment is a legitimate theoretical concern. The concept involved is of interest to academicians and others who have no specific interest in application. Second, the thrust for applying the techniques of mental health needs assessment has, until recently, come in large part from the requirements of the Community Mental Health Center program. Instead of letting the action of the marketplace determine the evolution of mental health facilities, federal requirements for documentation and evaluation influenced the evolution of mental health needs assessment methods.

Neither of these forces has created a methodology that easily meets a major current requirement of needs methodologies. Instead of region-wide, relatively expensive techniques, the necessity of satisfying certificate of need (CON) requirements has created a desire for mental health needs assessment technique with the following characteristics:

1. It must be portable, that is, there should be no requirement for data from an in-place, complex, ongoing data collection scheme established for the purpose of needs assessment.

2. The technique should be adaptable to the requirement of a one-shot assessment for a certificate-of-need application. Especially in the investment of private capital for new facilities, there is little likelihood of repeating the needs assessment.

Jack LaPatra, Ph.D., School of Health Systems, Georgia Institute of Technology, Atlanta.

3. Since the technique will be applied to one facility, it must be capable of dealing with a single service area that may be small.

4. The results of the assessment should include the prospective number of admissions in each treatment mode and length of stay.

5. The assessment and its result must be credible to a Health Systems Agency (HSA) review board that may be inexperienced, have particular technical biases, or is politically motivated.

In terms of what is available to do a mental health needs assessment, this is a tall order.

Summary of Existing Assessment Methodologies

In Table 1 the existing mental health needs assessment methodologies are summarized according to their ratings over the following dimensions: amount of data required, advantages, disadvantages, cost, skill level required, amount of effort required and quality of results. A simple rating of high, medium or low was assigned to each dimension of each methodology.

Practice

The most common assessment methodology is use rates. The popularity of use rates is a graphic example of a failure to follow this statement: "Statistical analysis cannot be a sufficient test of any model and the plausibility of the theoretical base is critical."

In a recent survey Bachrach [1] found research suggesting psychiatric bed use rates in the range of 0.2 to 3.75 beds per 1000 people — nearly a factor of 19 to 1. The difficulty is well-stated in the preface to her report:

> "The problem is a complex one since there are no generally applicable 'natural laws' for determining the ratio of such beds to population. Theoretical models for computing this ratio can be provided. However, such models require that incidence and prevalence rates for mental disorders, admission and release rates to psychiatric beds for persons with such disorders be known and that

Table 1. Mental Health Needs Assessment Methodology Summary

Method	*Amount of Data Required*	*Advantages*	*Disadvantages*	*Cost*	*Skill Level Required*	*Amount of Effort Required*	*Quality of Results*
Key informant	Medium	Medium	Medium	Low	Medium	Low	Low
Community forum	Low	Low	High	Low	Medium	Low	Low
Nominal group	Medium	High	Medium	Medium	Medium	Low	Medium
Use rates	Medium	Low	High	Medium	Low	High	Low
General surveys	High	Medium	Medium	High	Medium	High	Medium
Demographic social indicator	High	Medium	Medium	High	Medium	High	Medium
Ecological social indicator	High	Medium	Medium	High	High	High	Medium
Epidemiological survey	High	High	High	High	High	High	High

these rates and their trends can be determined and predicted reliably."

Unfortunately, research by Warheit and others [13] has shown that there is a wide gulf between the mental health needs of a community as determined by field prevalence surveys and the number of persons receiving mental health care in the same community.

Thus we see what is now a near-classic quandary, a field prevalence survey — a type of epidemiological survey — intends to measure need. Because such a survey is too expensive and complex for most people to mount, a proxy measure, use rates, is measured instead. But use rates are a demand measure and the theoretical connection between demand and need is unknown. If the connection between demand and need were known, there is little question that two significant variables that must be considered are time and location.

The situation and time specific requirement of mental health needs and demand assessment is what makes everything about this issue so complicated. The question which must be answered is: Where and how can I obtain the data in order to choose the most suitable use rate in the published range and in that way make the designated use rate a high-quality proxy measure of need?

I know of no HSA that has an answer to that question, and in its absence a locally decided use rate is selected. Often the midrange figure of 1.8 beds per 1000 people [1] is chosen. Tooth and Brooke [1] also estimate that the mental health beds will be used by 20% of short-term patients. These figures can be related to length of treatment modes and then (at least vaguely) to types of mental illness. This appears to be the only hint in the literature where research suggests indirectly what illness will occupy the beds determined by a use rate.

In summary, use rates can be influenced by the following factors: (1) treatment modes used by the local mental health professionals; (2) health consciousness of the local people and (3) number of mental health facilities available locally.

Recently we surveyed all HSAs to determine their approach to mental health needs assessment. We found that 67 of the 103 HSAs responding to the survey have yet to develop some form of planning for psychiatric beds. Most of these HSAs revealed that their inability to plan for psychiatric beds was due not only to a lack of expertise in mental health planning, but also because there were no apparent valid and reliable models to follow.

Eleven HSAs are trying to deal with the assessment problem by applying ratios that are used in planning general medical-surgical beds to psychiatric bed needs. Psychiatric beds cannot be discussed in the same context as general medical-surgical beds. There is not only a distinct difference between these types of beds, but there is also a major difference in the classification of psychiatric beds. The problem remains because they have not addressed psychiatric bed needs as a separate entity with its own unique set of problems.

The majority of the HSAs (22) that were attempting to discuss psychiatric bed needs as a separate issue were using planning methods that identified patterns of utilization as an indicator of need. They are facing the problem of not only dealing with changing patterns within the mental health system, but also the collection and analysis of the data necessary for decision making.

Finally, there were two HSAs that were attempting to incorporate variables that are correlated with mental illness into a model and develop an indicator of need.

Strategy

Based on the discussion to this point, the following strategy is proposed as a mental health needs assessment technique appropriate to the specified application. This approach is currently undergoing testing.

1. Utilize brief interviews (in person or telephone) with health professionals, psychiatrists, social service professionals and knowledgeable consumers to pick a Delphi panel.

2. Use the Delphi panel to determine:

a) Nominal group panel

b) Problem statement for nominal group

c) Other data

3. Run a "modified" nominal group process to acquire specific material and data needed for CON application.

Understanding of the above strategy requires basic knowledge of the Delphi and nominal group processes. In effect, the

Delphi is being used in advance of the nominal group to deal with the limitations of the nominal group. The Delphi process is used as a variant of a group decision-making activity to provide unique inputs to the nominal group. Both processes will require modification.

In effect, the Delphi method is used for soliciting and aggregating opinions on the broader initial issues involved in the application, while using the nominal group to compose solutions once having specific problems at hand.

Delphi

In Delphi, a carefully designed questionnaire is recirculated to the anonymous participants several times. In each successive round the questionnaire contains additional information about earlier responses and the degree of consensus reached to date. The continual feedback stimulates the responders to reevaluate their positions until a consensus is reached or until distinct positions have been identified. In effect, the Delphi process aims to aggregate the individual data into group data.

Nominal Group Process (NGP)

The NGP is an actual group meeting in which the objective of the study is interactively considered in the format of a question. Ideas regarding the question are shared in the presence of others and creative tension is stimulated by means of the presence of others, the silence and the evidence of activity. A series of structured round robins and votes aggregate the various members' judgments into a group decision.

Conclusion

The general difficulty with the "soft" mental health assessment techniques is the aggregation of the data. The combined sequential use of the Delphi panel and the nominal group resolves this difficulty. The power of the combination allows the identification of the need for special medical facilities from the need for general facilities.

References

1. Bachrach, L.L.: Psychiatric Bed Needs: An Analytical Review. DHEW Publication No. ADM 75-205, Washington, D.C., 1975.
2. Cohen, H.S.: Regulating health care facilities: The certificate-of-need process re-examined. Inquiry X:3-9, 1973.
3. Correia, E.: Public certification of need for health facilities. Am. J. Public Health 65 (3):260-265, 1975.
4. Rice, D.P. and Kleinman, J.C.: National health data for policy and planning. *In* Elinson, J. et al (eds.): Health Goals and Health Indicators: Policy, Planning, and Evaluation. Westview Press, 1977.
5. Huscani, B.A. and Neff, J.A.: The Mental Health Needs of a Rural Middle Tennessee County. Nashville, Tenn.:Tennessee State University, 1977.
6. Moore, W.S. and Block, H.B.: Estimating the demand for medical care. Inquiry IX:64-67, 1962.
7. Morris, H.J. (ed.): Determination of Need Methodologies. A report from the American Hospital Association, Chicago, Illinois, 1974.
8. Rosoff, A.J.: Health planning and certification of need under the new federal health planning act. Hosp. Admin. pp. 60-71, 1975.
9. Salkever, D.S. and Bice, T.W.: The impact of certificate-of-need controls on hospital investment. Health Society pp. 185-214, 1976.
10. Schwab, J.J. et al: Needs assessment methods for the community mental health center. Evaluation (2):64-76, 1975.
11. Schwab, J.J. and Warheit, G.J.: Evaluating southern mental health needs and services. J. Fla. Med. Assoc. 59(1):17-20, 1972.
12. Stuehler, G.: Certification of need — a systems analysis of Maryland's experience and plans. Am. J. Public Health 63(11):966-972, 1973.
13. Warheit, G.J.: Needs Assessment Approaches: Concepts and Methods. DHEW Publication No. (ADM) 77-472, Washington, D.C., 1977.
14. Whitten, F.D.: Playing the numbers planning game. Hosp. Financing Management 39:29-32, 1978.

Role of Police in the Emergency Medical Services System

Justin A. Myrick, Ph.D.

There has been much discussion of using public safety agency personnel as part of the emergency medical system of a community. Much of this discussion has been prompted by the mandate of the Emergency Medical Services Systems Act of 1973 (PL 93-154) stating that effective utilization of appropriate public safety agencies should be obtained. The Health Systems Research Center of Georgia Institute of Technology recently completed a two-year research project funded by the National Center for Health Services Research (R 18 HS 01767) to evaluate performance of the police officer as a first responder to medical emergencies within an existing Emergency Medical Services (EMS) system. The research setting was DeKalb County, Georgia, one of the central counties within the Atlanta metropolitan area.

The primary responder to medical emergencies in DeKalb County is the DeKalb County Fire Department operating modern ambulance units based in neighborhood fire stations but possessing a county-wide central emergency medical phone number. The DeKalb County Fire Department and the DeKalb County Police Department have a verbal agreement to notify each other as emergency medical calls are received. This is accomplished by a ring-down dedicated phone line connecting the dispatchers. Each organization, therefore, responds to each emergency situation.

The DeKalb County police officers complete a 40-hour first aid training program as part of the DeKalb Police Academy. As an indicator of importance placed upon first aid, this is one of

---

Justin A. Myrick, Ph.D., Associate Professor, School of Health Systems, Georgia Institute of Technology, Atlanta.

only two sections of the training program in which a passing grade must be obtained.

Overall Purpose

The overall purpose of this research project was to evaluate the performance of medically trained police officers serving as rapid response resources in conjunction with an EMS system. This routine response of police officers to medical emergencies for the purpose of administering first aid procedures prior to the arrival of an ambulance was referred to in the project as the medical aid vehicle (MAV) concept. This purpose was pursued through the following objectives:

- To analyze an existing police trauma-management training program for the purpose of describing medical skills being taught to participants in the program.
- To describe a task, or group of tasks, from the existing training program, which should be performed for specific, individual medical emergencies.
- To determine the frequency with which police perform specific MAV tasks and other nonmedical tasks in a functional MAV environment.
- To assess the relationship between police performance of MAV skills and performance of "traditional" duties associated with law enforcement.
- To measure behavioral attitudes and perceptions of police and the public in regard to the police MAV concept.

The use of police in a first-responder role appears to have several advantages. Some of the advantages which are intuitively appealing are:

- Police department vehicles are more numerous than fire combat vehicles and therefore should be capable of quicker response.
- Police vehicles are usually in motion and manned at the time they are dispatched. Fire combat

vehicles are usually stationary and unmanned at the time they are dispatched.

- Patrol cars appear to be more maneuverable than fire trucks and should be capable of quicker response if congested, narrow, or curved roads must be traveled.
- Patrol cars are frequently observed at the scene of a medical emergency prior to the arrival of a fire combat team or an ambulance, indicating that police vehicles routinely respond to many medical emergencies.
- The use of police in this capacity appears to require little additional resources in order to perform this role effectively.

Thus, the use of police in responding to emergencies has great potential in improving the EMS system. The extent to which that potential could be realized was of great interest to the study.

Major Findings

The research project specifically examined the MAV concept as it operates in the DeKalb County (Georgia) Police Department, and hence all of the results are not necessarily applicable to other situations. However, the many commonalities associated with law enforcement agencies imply that much of the research is generalizable to other situations. The overall purpose of the research was to examine the basic foundation of the MAV concept, namely, to provide quick first response to medical emergencies using existing police resources. Questions of particular interest to decision-makers considering implementation of the MAV concept which were addressed during the course of the project include the following:

- Will utilization of police officers as first responders provide quicker response to medical emergencies?
- Will police officers perform first aid given the opportunity and training?
- Will police officers accept the first aid role as part of their overall police role?

- Will there be a conflict between performance of first aid duties and performance of traditional law enforcement duties?
- How should such a program be coordinated within a community in order to maximize its benefits?
- What are the resource requirements associated with the implementation of the MAV concept?
- Will the public accept this MAV role and be supportive of it?

The answers to these questions have implications regarding not only the overall feasibility of the MAV concept, but also have significant bearing on a number of operational considerations relevant to successful implementation of the MAV concept.

In general, the research has indicated the MAV concept is indeed feasible and can be operated with considerable success within the community. Some of the specifics associated with this general conclusion are summarized below.

Response to Medical Emergencies

With respect to the quickness of response, it was found that police typically can and do arrive on the scene prior to the arrival of an ambulance. Overall mean response time for police was 5.2 minutes, whereas the mean for EMS was 7.2 minutes. Moreover, the amount of time on the scene prior to the arrival of other assistance is significant in terms of whether first aid was rendered. Since the police already routinely respond to traffic accidents and violence-related incidents in which first aid is required, and since they can be first to arrive on the scene, the performance of first aid by the officer is indeed important. In the study of approximately 4,000 cases, based upon response time data and assuming a simultaneous notification of the police and EMS, the police could have been on the scene prior to EMS in 66% of the cases. However, in only 36% of the cases did police actually arrive prior to EMS. This appears to be due to dispatch delays which are occurring in the dispatch centers. These delays need to be corrected before the police can be as effective as possible.

Performance of First Aid

With respect to performance, the amount of first aid delivered by the officers in the study group was uniformly low. Of 1,348 cases in which police arrived prior to EMS, first aid was performed in only 478 cases. This appeared to be related to the availability of highly sophisticated EMS resources in the study site. For a high number of nonserious cases, the police tended to wait for ambulance personnel to take care of less serious emergencies, but the police tended to render care immediately in life-threatening situations. The study showed a significantly higher level of performance for the more serious emergencies.

The First Aid Role

Acceptance of the first aid role as part of the police officer's overall duties is an important aspect to consider. Behavioral implications may possibly be the most critical factors to consider when implementing the MAV concept. Police officers must be motivated to perform first aid and must consider emergency medical services as part of their primary police role if the MAV concept is to be successful. Behavioral surveys conducted during the project indicated that the police in the study group supported the MAV concept and were willing to perform basic first aid. However, this attitude was not uniformly shared by all officers.

Highlights of the behavioral study included the following points:

> There was no perceived conflict between officers and EMTs. The officers did not view their work as an infringement upon EMTs. The officers also did not agree that first aid creates too much work. There was also a strong feeling that police first aid provides more rapid first aid care and better emergency care. There was strong disagreement with the proposition that only EMTs should deliver emergency care. There was likewise strong agreement that the idea of police rendering first aid is a good one. First aid training was also strongly felt to be a real personal asset which was not limited to the job. While

officers were not sure that their ability to give first aid could be used more than it currently is, there is decidedly strong agreement with the proposition that police cars ought to be dispatched at the same time as ambulances to a medical emergency.

Conflicts With Other Duties

Performance of first aid tasks did not appear to be significantly related to a conflict with traditional law enforcement duties. This may be due in part to the notion that the police officer's first responsibility is to the victim, regardless of whether the police officer is medically trained. Thus, training police officers in first aid gives the officer the capability to effectively handle situations which he frequently encounters in conjunction with his traditional law enforcement duties.

Community Coordination

It was found that interagency communication and cooperation are very important aspects in implementing the MAV concept. Conflict between different agencies in rendering EMS can have a pronounced effect on the effectiveness of the MAV concept. In addition, when different agencies are responsible for responding to emergencies, it is essential that responsibilities be specified in detail and that all agencies are aware of their respective roles. The study site demonstrated some communication barriers between the two agencies regarding the specific role that each is to play. This is resulting in dispatch delays which reduce the effectiveness of the concept.

Resource Requirements

With regard to resource requirements associated with implementation of the MAV concept, delivery of first aid was not perceived as being "extra work" by the officer. In addition, it was found that in order to provide the basic stabilizing care in a first-responder capacity, the police officer needs little equipment. A good first aid kit in the trunk of each police vehicle is a valuable asset but was not used heavily. A training program at the level of 40 hours appears to be appropriate and should not overly tax the training resources of the department. The program, however, will require considerable training time for departments having many officers to train. Another consideration is periodic retraining of officers needed in order to insure that the officers maintain their first aid skills. Refresher training at six-month intervals should be planned in order to review the basic stabilization skills.

Public Acceptance

A structured telephone survey of public emergency aid-seeking behavior conducted during the study period revealed that in approximately 10% to 15% of medical emergencies, the public is likely to call the police first for assistance. This percentage is 25% to 40% for emergency conditions requiring police involvement such as vehicle accidents involving injuries. The public thus views the role of a policeman as a resource in medical emergencies and is especially true for situations in which the police normally become involved.

Conclusion

This project has shown that police officers are very important in providing first-responder capability in DeKalb County. With greater understanding and cooperation by all agencies involved, the first-responder role could and should become even more valuable. Nothing has been found that would indicate this same effective emergency response system could not be incorporated in other urban/suburban settings.

Impact of Gratuitousness on Prescribed Medicine Use by the Elderly

Jacques Tremblay, M.D.

Several social programs have been designed in the past to help satisfy unmet needs in health care systems. As such, drug programs have been implemented in several countries [1]. The aim of these programs is to improve access to prescribed medicines [1, 2], an essential component of current care [1, 3]. Prescribed medicines (PM) were thus made available without charge (gratuitousness) to those who benefit from the program (beneficiaries). The object of this paper is to examine the impact of gratuitousness on PM consumption behavior. The Quebec Drug Program and its elderly beneficiaries will be used for this purpose.

Several reviews of the literature on consumption of PM have been made in the past [4-6], with a minor emphasis placed on the impact of drug programs [6, 7]. Consumption of PM has previously been measured using two methods. The first method establishes utilization of PM by the analysis of dispensed prescriptions in pharmacy records [4]. This first approach has the advantage of using written, thus "harder" data sources, while acquisition rather than actual medicine-taking behavior is addressed. The second method establishes use of PM by collecting consumer statements on actual medicine-taking behavior. The term "use study" is proposed here to distinguish this type of research from prescription analysis. While based on

---

Jacques Tremblay, M.D., School of Pharmacy, Laval University, Quebec, Canada.

This research was performed under a national health scholarship (Canada #6605-1370-48).

"softer" data sources, this approach of use studies has been noted for its ability to produce internally consistent results [8]. There is the advantage of directly addressing medicine-taking behavior. Furthermore, home medicine cabinet storage and medicine-taking by others are excluded from measurement of consumption in use studies.

Neither utilization nor use studies have yet established clearly the impact of drug programs on PM consumption, contrary to statements made previously [6, 7]. Six utilization studies [9-14] have dealt with drug program impact on consumption of PM. Their conclusions are very contrasting. Three studies *showed an increase* in prescription utilization following drug program introduction [9-11], while three *failed to report this increase* [12-14]. All six studies suffer from selection biases, which may account for their inability to reach comparable conclusions. Thus, a clear picture of drug program impact is difficult to discern from utilization studies.

Two use studies have been unable to resolve this controversy. A major descriptive use study by the World Health Organization [8] established use of medicines, among other types of care, in seven different countries. A subsequent analysis of this data focused on the Baltimore area [15] and showed that those who paid none or only some of their medicine cost (under some drug program) were *not any more likely* to be users of PM than those who paid for all costs (not under a program), while non- and partial payers were contrastingly *more likely* to be users of morbidity-related PM than payers. A second use study attempted to assess the impact of the Quebec Drug Program on medicine use in a rural population [16]. This report observed no impact on total family medicine use, but failed to take into account such factors as family size or major determinants of PM. These characteristics would be morbidity, age, sex and medical services utilization [8]. Thus, the conflicting findings regarding the impact of drug programs on consumption of PM are evident, whether this impact is assessed indirectly by utilization studies or more directly by use studies. In order to shed more light on this question, the present study was undertaken in the context of the Quebec Drug Program. This program will now be briefly presented.

The province of Quebec has a population of 6 million, of which half a million are 65 years or older [17]. In 1961, hospital care became free for all Quebec residents. Ten years later, National Health Insurance came into effect, such as to insure medical services coverage. In 1972, the Quebec Drug Program was implemented to improve access to medicinal care for those in need. Welfare recipients were first eligible, followed in 1974 by recipients of the federal Program of Monthly Guaranteed Income Supplement [18-21]. The latter are 65 years or older, earn $2,500 Canadian per capita per year, or $4,500 Canadian per couple per year. In 1976, elderly beneficiaries of the Quebec Drug Program could account for 64% of the Quebec elderly [17, 22]. In October 1977, all of Quebec elderly became eligible for the drug program, regardless of income [23]. All costs for PM are covered by the Quebec Drug Program when listed in a formulary. This list of medicines is established and reviewed every six months by a pharmacology committee, based on product quality. Over-the-counter drugs are not covered by the program.

A rapidly increasing investment of public funds has been allotted to this program. Cost per eligible per year rose from $49 Canadian in 1974 to $70 two years later. In 1976, $51 million was allotted to this program alone, representing about 12% of the $441 million Canadian needed for coverage of medical services in Quebec [20, 22]. In a cost-containment perspective, such an investment has raised the question of drug program impact on beneficiary consumption behavior. In this perspective, two hypotheses were formulated for the present study: first, that elderly Quebec Program beneficiaries would report a statistically significant higher use of PM than nonbeneficiaries; second, that a longer period of benefit among beneficiaries would be associated with a statistically significant higher reported use of PM. The more direct use study approach was chosen.

The 1976 provincial electoral list, from the population living in a suburban section of a 500,000 urban and mostly francophone agglomeration, was modified by removing individuals who reported their residence as an institution or an age under 64. A simple random sample of 80 persons was drawn from this modified list. These persons accounted for 8% of the noninstitutionalized elderly in the study area. In August 1977, a female interviewer made home visits to the selected persons, presenting herself as an employee in a university research project. She carried out an interview with those who gave consent and met eligibility criteria. To be eligible, subjects were 65 years or older at the date of interview, lived outside of any institution and were free from invalidity, scoring "A" on the ADL scale [24].

The interview was structured and conducted in two parts. The first part established study eligibility, age, sex, Quebec Drug Program beneficiary status, duration of this benefit among beneficiaries and PM use in the 48 hours preceding interview. The second part included an inventory of the home medicine cabinet, which will not be reported here. Interview data were recorded on route sheets. The interviewer was unaware of the hypotheses being tested to prevent interviewer biases. French formulation of the PM use question was adapted from the WHO study [8]. The English translation would be: "In the last two days, did you take any medicine prescribed for you by a doctor? If so, how many different ones did you take?" Medical services utilization level, a major determinant of PM use [8], was also obtained by a record linkage method which allows protection of confidentiality. The number of visits performed by general practitioners on an ambulatory basis over a period of six months, from April to September 1977, was established by the staff of the Quebec Health Insurance Board. The medical claims file served as a data source. Record linkage between interview data and claims data was done in a coded form through a third party at the time of data analysis. This record linkage method will not be reported here.

Data analysis consisted of a test of both hypotheses with analysis of variance (ANOVA), using a standard option from the SPSS package [25]. ANOVA was designed to take into account the determinants of PM use and was itself performed in two steps. A first step involved screening for both hypotheses, without regard to medical services utilization. Only when such a screening confirmed an hypothesis would it be retested using the record linkage method. Use of PM served as the criterion (dependent variable) in all cases. For the screening of the first hypothesis, age, sex and Drug Program beneficiary status were used as factors (independent variables). For the screening of the second, beneficiary status was replaced by duration of benefit in completed years, and analysis limited to beneficiaries. The final step of ANOVA was to be performed if the hypothesis resisted screening, after addition of the medical services utilization factor with record linkage. All factors were subjected to a dichotomous classification process prior to analysis, as will be shown later. A multiple classification analysis [25] completed each ANOVA in order to assess the percentage of criterion variation explained by each factor and by the overall analytical model.

Of the original sample of 80, 49 elderly completed the interview (61%). The distribution of subjects by age, by sex and by drug program beneficiary status did not differ significantly from the 1976 Quebec population distribution, as tested by Chi-square, at the 5% level [17, 22].

The first ANOVA screening for the first hypothesis failed to show any significant main effect ($p > 0.50$). The second step of ANOVA was not performed and the first hypothesis is not supported. The first ANOVA screening for the second hypothesis behaved much differently, since joint main effects reached a high significance. The second ANOVA step was performed, using the medical services utilization factor with record linkage. Record linkage was successful for all beneficiaries. Results of this ANOVA are presented in Table 1. It can be seen that the classification of subjects for each ANOVA factor resulted in an appropriate sample partitioning. Joint main effects reached a high significance level ($p < 0.001$), but only the main effects of duration of benefit were significant individually ($p < 0.001$). Only one two-way interaction, between sex and medical services utilization, reached significance ($p < 0.01$), but not jointly with other interactions. Multiple classification analysis established that the analytical model accounted for 51% of criterion variation. Other multiple classification analysis scores are not given here, since interaction tends to make direct interpretation difficult [25]. In conclusion, the second hypothesis is strongly supported by the above results.

Before discussing results, some attention should be given to two assumptions which were made in this study. It was first assumed that ANOVA had sufficient robustness despite a lack

Table 1. ANOVA Results. Use of Prescribed Medicines by Duration of Benefit, Age, Sex and Medical Services Utilization (n = 35)

Factor	*Category*	*Number of Subjects in Category*	*Value of Factor in Category*	*F-Value**
Duration of benefit	1	15	0, 1, 2 years	34.757†
	2	20	3, 4, 5 years	
Age	1	23	65-74 years	1.190‡
	2	12	75 or more years	
Sex	1	12	Male	1.668‡
	2	23	Female	
Utilization of medical services	1	24	No services used	1.976‡
	2	11	One or more service used	

*Three-way and two-way interactions do not reach significance at the 5% level, except one between sex and utilization of medical services. ($F = 9.494$, $p < 0.01$)

†$p < 0.001$

‡$p > 0.15$

of normality in the distribution of ANOVA variables. Support for this first assumption may be found elsewhere [26]. Second, it was assumed that a natural tendency did not already exist in the Quebec aged population, such that early registration would have systematically occurred among higher users of PM, which would partially account for the present findings. This second assumption seems reasonable when examining the corollary that any systematic tendency among higher users of PM would be associated with the characteristics of higher users of PM described in seven countries [8]. The characteristics would be a presence of morbidity, female sex, higher age and utilization of medical services. The three last factors were taken into account by ANOVA. Thus, to maintain validity, it is necessary that only morbidity be accounted for. Since medical services utilization may serve as a proxy measure for morbidity (D. L. Rabin, personal communication, February 7, 1978), it was at least partially taken into account by ANOVA. Second, since persons with invalidity and/or institutional status were excluded from the present study, their higher morbidity (and higher medicine consumption) were also eliminated. Therefore, it is necessary to assume only that the preselection criterion has been sufficient to control the effects of morbidity. The results of the present study seem to corroborate this assumption, since the mean reported use of PM (1.35 PM per subject) was slightly lower than that reported for the neighboring region of northern Vermont (1.46 PM per subject) in the WHO study [8]. Thus, the presence of exceptional morbidity in this sample seems highly unlikely, and support for this assumption may be found.

Interpretation of present results must also be made in the context of a limitation. Because of budgetary and time constraints, this study was limited to a small sample size. Care should be taken in attempting to generalize the present findings to the entire Quebec elderly population, even though Chi-square tests indicated that the sample, with regard to age, sex and beneficiary status distribution, was not significantly different from the Quebec elderly population.

In view of these comments, an interpretation can be put forward to account for the present findings. The first hypothesis was not supported, since use of PM by beneficiaries was not significantly higher than use by nonbeneficiaries. Since beneficiaries at the time of the study were at a lower end of an economic classification with a per capita income under $2,500, as discussed earlier, this first finding implies that there was no difference in PM use by two contrasting income categories. This corroborates earlier findings in the Baltimore area [15]. It is proposed that differences in use related to income would have existed prior to the introduction of the Program, but have been obliterated by the removal of financial barriers to PM acquisition. A similar phenomenon was described for medical services utilization under National Health Insurance [27]. This would also imply that the Quebec Drug Program has been *successful in raising accessibility* to medicinal care.

The second hypothesis has been supported, while accounting for the effects of major determinants of PM use. There was a tendency among beneficiaries to report significantly higher use of PM with increasing benefit duration. The current analytical model was also powerful in accounting for half the variation in criterion. The increase of PM use as a *direct consequence of gratuitousness* under a drug program is an interpretation which fully accounts for the current findings. Furthermore, the time-section addressed by the study (five years) points to the possibility of a *long-term effect* on beneficiaries.

Further implications of this impact may be considered if it is assumed that the impact of drug programs extends to psychotropics (affecting the function of the central nervous system) as well as other PM. From 1972 to 1975, psychotropics constituted one third of PM dispensed under the Quebec Drug Program [21]. Most of these psychotropics were benzodiazepines, such as chlordiazepoxide and diazepam [23]. Since benzodiazepines should generally not be used for periods exceeding two weeks [28], serious consideration should be given to the inappropriateness of such consumption. Strategies should be developed in a cost-containment perspective. One option would be to limit drug coverage under programs, such as to exclude benzodiazepines. Restrictions on an already granted privilege might prove a major obstacle to this first option. A second option would direct Health Education at diminishing inappropriate medicine use. Psychotropic medicines, such as benzodiazepines, could be chosen as a target. For this option, further understanding in the area of the determinants of psychotropic medicine use must first be reached, so that Health Education be oriented in a meaningful way. Then, a rigorous evaluation could be conducted, both to establish program efficiency (in cost-benefit terms) and efficacy (reduction in use). It is to be hoped that such interventions, if adequately planned and evaluated, will succeed in limiting unwanted effects of a drug program.

References

1. Drug Coverage Under National Health Insurance: The Policy Options. National Center for Health Services Research. Department of Health, Education, and Welfare Publication Number (HRA) 77-3189. Washington, 1977.
2. Tremblay, J.: Evaluation Research and Drug Coverage Under National Health Insurance. Unpublished communication to staff. National Center for Health Services Research, Hyattsville, Md., May 22, 1978.
3. Hemminki, E.: The role of prescriptions in therapy. Med. Care 13:150, 1975.

4. Rabin, D.L.: Use of medicines: A review of prescribed and non-prescribed medicine use. Med. Care Rev. 29:668, 1972.
5. Rabin, D.L. and Bush, P.J.: The use of medicines: Historical trends and international comparisons. Int. J. Health Serv. 4:61, 1974.
6. Rabin, D.L.: Prescribed and nonprescribed medicine use. *In* Wertheimer, A.I. and Bush, P.J. (eds.): Perspectives on Medicines in Society. Hamilton, Ill.:Drug Intelligence Publications, 1977, p. 55.
7. Donabedian, A.: Benefits in Medical Care Programs. Cambridge: Harvard University Press, 1976, p. 62.
8. Health Care: An International Study. Kohn, R. and White, K.L. (eds.). New York:Oxford University Press, 1976, pp. xviii, 223-227, 487, 519.
9. Greenlick, M.R. and Darsky, B.J.: A comparison of general drug utilization in a metropolitan community with utilization under a drug prepayment plan. Am. J. Public Health 58:2121, 1968.
10. Smith, M.C. and Garner, D.D.: Effects of a Medicaid program on prescription drug availability and acquisition. Med. Care 12:571, 1974.
11. Weeks, H.A.: Changes in prescription drug utilization after the introduction of a prepaid drug insurance program. J. Am. Pharm. Assoc. NS 13:205, 1973.
12. Johnson, R.E., Campbell, W.H. and Azevedo, D.J.: Examining the drug utilization and expenditures of a medically indigent population. Inquiry 15:38, 1978.
13. Rabin, D.L., Bush, P.J. and Fuller, N.A.: Drug prescription rates before and after enrollment of a Medicaid population in an HMO. Public Health Rep. 93:16, 1978.
14. Yesalis, C.E. III and Bonnet, P.D.: The effect of duration of membership in a prepaid group health plan on the utilization of services. Med. Care 14:1024, 1976.
15. Rabin, D.L. and Bush, P.J.: Who's using prescribed medicines? Drug Health Care 3:89, 1976.
16. Beaudoin, R., Lemay, Y. and Leblanc, J.B.: Etude de la consommation de médicaments dans un milieu rural québecois. Médicaments d'aujourd'hui 1,4, 1977.
17. 1976 Census of Canada. Population: Demographic Characteristics. Five-Year Age Groups. Statistics Canada Publication Number 92-823. Ottawa, 1978.
18. Old Age Security Act. RS., chapters 0-6, Government of Canada, Ottawa, 1977.
19. Morreale, J.C.: The cost of national health insurance: The Province of Québec. Inquiry 14:330, 1977.
20. Statistiques Annuelles 1974. Régie de l'Assurance-Maladie du Québec, Québec, 1975.
21. Statistiques Annuelles 1975. Régie de l'Assurance-Maladie du Québec, Québec, 1976.
22. Statistiques Annuelles 1976. Régie de l'Assurance-Maladie du Québec, Québec, 1977.

23. Unpublished Data. Régie de l'Assurance-Maladie du Québec, Québec, 1978.
24. Katz, S., Ford, A.B., Moskowitz, R.W. et al: Studies of illness in the aged. The Index of ADL: A standardized measure of biological and psychosocial function. JAMA 185:914, 1963.
25. Kim, J.O. and Kohout, F.J.: Analysis of variance and covariance: Subprograms ANOVA and ONEWAY. *In* Nie, N.H. et al (eds.): SPSS Statistical Package for the Social Sciences. Montréal:McGraw-Hill, 1975, p. 398.
26. Dunn, O.J. and Clark, V.A.: Applied Statistics: Analysis of Variance and Regression. New York:Wiley, 1974, p. 347.
27. National Health Insurance: Can We Learn From Canada? Andreopoulos, S. (ed.). New York:Wiley, 1975, p. 117.
28. Sellers, E.M.: Clinical pharmacology and therapeutics of benzodiazepines. Can. Med. Assoc. J. 118:1533, 1978.

Profiling for Efficacy in Long-Range Clinical Trials

Turkan Kumbaraci Gardenier, Ph.D.

Introduction

Clinical decisions often involve classifying a patient into either receiving benefit from the treatment prescribed, showing no change in status or worsening as a function of time. Azen and Afifi [1] presented analyses of this kind involving a Bayesian approach for time-dependent observations. Karacan et al [2] and Yeng and Hursch [3] used semi-Markovian models to depict the sequence of continuous clinical data. The life-table model with multivariate criteria has been used by Cox [4] and applied to successive observations.

Sequential procedures in clinical studies have often used group sequential designs where an equal number of patients are tested on two medications and where the hypothesis tested, at each stage, is whether the two medications are equally effective. Darwin [5] suggested the use of a derived score with Trinomial characteristics (1, 0, −1) to compare paired observations on successive evaluations. Operating characteristics of the binomial distribution for group sequential designs have been presented by Armitage [6], Bross [7] and Elfring and Schultz [8].

None of the above formulations, however, deal with time-series data for a specific patient and the query of how long medication may continue until a decision is made, with sufficient statistical reliability, as to whether the patient has shown improvement or worsening due to medication. The objective of this paper is to introduce the framework for decisions of this type.

Turkan Kumbaraci Gardenier, Ph.D., Adjunct Professor of Biostatistics, Columbia University and President, Teka Trends, Inc., Washington, D.C.

Trinomial Framework

The Trinomial framework is reminiscent of the use of control charts in quality control. Tolerance limits are specified which provide bounds for satisfactory operation. If observed values exceed the "bounds," i.e., the upper and lower limits of the control chart, they are considered unacceptable. If a sufficient number of "unacceptable" observations are observed successively, the system is considered out of control which triggers a mechanism for analysis of causes for such deviation. Attribute sampling methods using the Trinomial and contour diagrams for decision-making have been presented by Bray and Lyon [9]. Credeur [10] analyzed convergence criteria with estimation decisions using incomplete Trinomial data.

Although control charts are usually encountered in industrial engineering settings, the framework would be useful for clinical evaluation decisions. Consider, for example, measurements for blood glucose for a diabetic patient, diastolic blood pressure for a patient with hypertension or measurements for serum cholesterol for a patient with hyperlipidemia. If normal limits for these variables have been predetermined, a patient's successive measurements may follow a pattern such as that depicted in Figure 1.

The "normal" range in Figure 1 shows the region of acceptability; regions outside this limit show either extreme of the "unacceptable." That is, the +1 range would indicate hyperactivity, such as elevated blood glucose levels, hypertension of hyperlipidemia; the −1 range would indicate abnormally low levels of the respective measurements.

Furthermore, we may conjecture that if we were to trace the observations, we could derive another index based upon *successive* observations and the *switching* patterns in the transition. An illustration is given in Figure 2. The evaluation

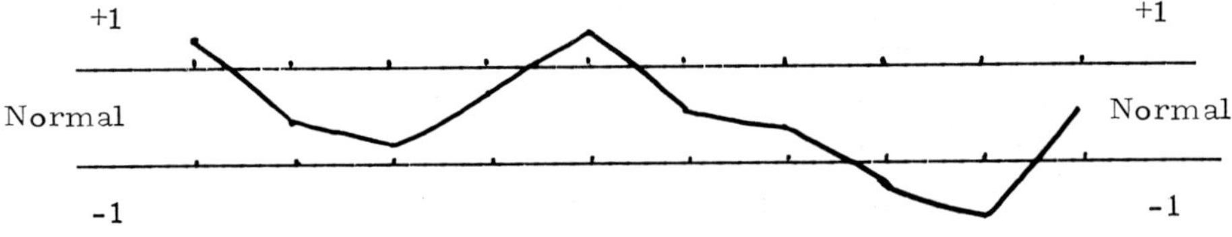

FIG. 1. Preliminary trichotomizations of successive measurements.

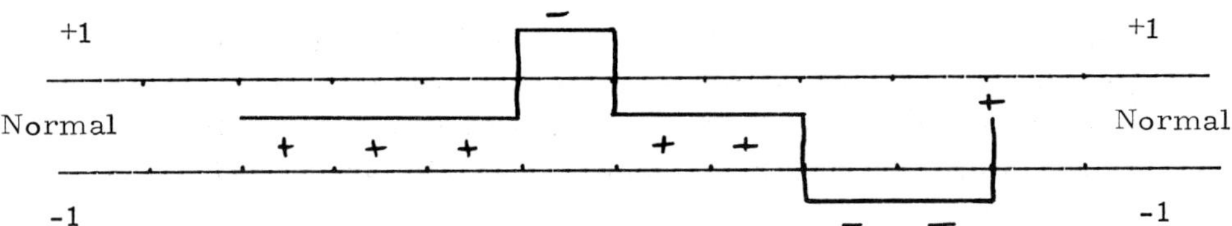

FIG. 2. Transition index based on changes in status in the Trinomial.

scheme is contingent upon whether the system is *maintained* at normal (within the bounds of control limits), whether there is a switch from *outside to within* normal limits, or whether there is a switch in the reverse direction. Thus, it is based upon *transition switches* in the Trinomial status. As will be observed in Figure 2, there is one less transition than number of successive observations.

An evaluation or weighting scheme superimposed upon the possibilities in the pattern in switches may be designed; two examples used by the present author are shown in Figure 3. In the first, maintenance within normal bounds is evaluated positively (+1), any switch from normal to outside normal

Switching Pattern	Scheme 1	Scheme 2
Normal --> Normal	+1	+1
Normal --> +1	-1	-1
Normal --> -1	-1	-1
+1 --> Normal	+1	+1
+1 --> +1	-1	0
+1 --> -1	-1	0
-1 --> Normal	+1	+1
-1 --> +1	-1	0
-1 --> -1	-1	0

FIG. 3. Two alternative evaluation schemes in transitions.

limits or remaining outside control limits is evaluated as (−1); a switch from either extreme to normal status is evaluated as (+1). The second alternative scheme presents a further modification in that maintenance outside control limits is weighted as *0*.

Criteria for Stopping Rules

Relative probabilities derived from the frequency of occurrence of +1, 0, and −1 in the evaluation scheme may be used in the determination of a null hypothesis under Neyman-Pearson formulations. Let us assume that if the prescribed medication has no effect, the probability of each transition state will be equal and that the transition states are independently distributed in successive observations. Therefore, the relative frequency of each of the three transition categories in the possible evaluation schema in Figure 3 may be used as the basis for the null hypothesis. A model analogous to estimation of reliability of subsystems in series may be used to determine the acceptability levels of consistent successive occurrence of improvement or worsening in patient status. The algorithm would be based upon p raised to the k power, where p denotes the probability of improvement (+1) or worsening (−1) and k denotes the number of follow-up periods. The level of significance would be $1\text{-}p^k$ in successive consistently occurring observations. Table 1 is based upon these formulations and the number of follow-up observations for significance levels of .05 and .01, respectively.

It will be observed as a result of scanning Table 1 that an observation of consistent improvement after the fourth or fifth visit would enable the clinician to conclude that medication is

Table 1. Successive Indices of Improvement or Worsening for Significance Levels of .05 and .01

	Follow-Up Periods				
	3	*4*	*5*	*6*	
Improvement	.109	.036	.012	.004	$\alpha = .05$
Worsening	.048	.011	.002	.005	$\alpha = .01$

producing an improvement over prior status. On the other hand, an observation of consistent deterioration in status after the third or fourth follow-up time may lead to the necessity to change the medication administered or to drop the patient from the clinical trial. Removing patients from the trial yields decreased total costs. The table also implies that decisions relating to worsening can be reached earlier than those relating to improvement. The nature of the transition matrix and evaluation scheme could be changed from trial to trial, modifying the stopping rules. Inputs to these decisions may be obtained from prototype analyses of successive patient status and overall trends shown as a result of administering the medication.

Comparisons between two active medications or medication and placebo may also be made by tabulating the number of patients who have shown consistent improvement and consistent deterioration in status as a function of clinical trial length. Table 2 shows an example of this type of comparison in a study where 80 patients were randomized into Medications A and B, 40 in each group.

In Table 2 two subtables are displayed: the first for patients who have shown consistent improvement in status by follow-up period i; the second subtable displays the similar results for patients with consistent deterioration in status. Statistical procedures for contingency table analysis, such as the Chi-square test, may be applied to the data for significance testing of relative efficacy between Medication A and B.

Table 2. Across-Medication Comparisons To Evaluate Group Effects

	Sequence of Evaluations on Follow-Up Visits				
	2	*3*	*4*	*5*	*6*
	Consistent Improvements				
Medication A	20	10	5	1	0
Medication B	10	8	4	0	0
	Consistent Deteriorations				
Medication A	4	3	1	0	0
Medication B	12	8	5	4	4

CTSS: The Cumulative Transitional State Score

This method of scoring successive clinical data has been applied by the present author to clinical data and has been found successful as a method for summarizing patient status in long-term studies. In ongoing applications the total index generated has been referred to as CTSS, a cumulative transitional state score, since it is based upon transitions or changes in status in successive evaluations.

Validation analyses are presently being conducted in order to evaluate the relative efficacy of CTSS as compared with other statistical measures. One of these analyses has involved correlating, through the use of product moment correlation coefficients, values for CTSS with the arithmetic mean of observations over successive visits, with the range in values and with a dichotomized Binomial evaluation of patient status. The Binomial evaluation involved characterizing, clinically, patient status as "normal" or outside the normal range regardless of whether the values were abnormally too high or too low. This method was formerly suggested by reviewers of the proposed CTSS methodology since more extensive publications and research exist using the Binomial distribution. Table 3 shows the product moment correlations results for these various indices. The data set consisted of data for four successive evaluations of enzyme levels obtained from 35 outpatients. As additional indices, the initial value of the observations and the sum of first and second, and the sum of the first three observations were used for each patient. The results are revealing in terms of the correlation in time series or autocor-

Table 3. Correlations Among Several Indices for Time-Dependent Values

	Binominal	*CTSS*
Initial Value	.659	.206
Range	–.043	.322
1 & 2	.726	.442
1 & 2 & 3	.749	.423
Arithmetic Mean	.833	.602

relation in the successive values of the covariance of the time-indexed values with the initial observation.

An evaluation of the data in Table 3 shows four interesting facets of CTSS. First, it correlates with initial observation to a lower degree than a Binomial summary measure, .206 versus .659. If one is interested in deriving an improvement measure, less covariance with initial observation is preferable. Second, there *is* a correlation with the range in observations with CTSS, but not with the Binomial. It may be worthwhile to note the degree of fluctuation in summarized successive values; thus, CTSS would be preferred from this standpoint. Third, measures of autocorrelation, as depicted by the third and fourth lines of Table 3, reveal that the Binomial is affected to a higher degree by autocorrelation than does CTSS — the correlations are in the .40 range rather than in the .70s. Fourth, the Binomial correlates higher with the arithmetic mean than does CTSS, implying, perhaps, that other components of "change" are being measured by the latter index.

Discussion

The procedure described above may be used in many settings where continuous data may be dichotomized or trichotomized. In previous reports the present author had discussed the applications of this procedure with clinical and industrial data [11-14]. The first applications of this scoring technique were with measurements in gastrointestinal symptoms. It has recently found applications as a generalized framework for monitoring. Particularly in clinical settings it enables evaluation of the trace in status for a particular patient without recourse to a comparison of only two points, the baseline and final value.

Elfring and Schultz [8] have used the Trinomial in group sequential designs. When transition probabilities are considered in profiling analysis, any function generates the Trinomial. This is because the next value, as compared with a prior value, is either equal to it, higher or lower. Thus the method has applications to any sequence function and time-series related data.

The Trinomial has two distinct uses in tracing patient status over time: First, it classifies each observed value as "above normal" (+1), "normal" (*0*), and "below normal" (−1), thereby explicitly specifying patient status at any point in time. Profiling of patient status across variables becomes easier, since the clinician or statistician does not need to refer to normal ranges. Second, the *transition* states of "improvement" (+1), "no change" (0) and "worsening" (−1) generate another index for evaluating *changes* in state in addition to describing states of health. The method thus provides a dual index of efficacy for use in long-range clinical trials. The starting and ending points for evaluation may be changed by the user, enabling summary comparisons between any two time periods.

References

1. Azen, S.P. and Afifi, A.A.: Asymptotic and small sample behavior of estimated Bayes rules for classifying time-dependent observations. Biometrics 28:989-998, 1972.
2. Karacan, I., Williams, R.L., Salis, P. and Hursch, C.J.: Approaches to the evaluation and treatment of insomnia. Psychosomatics 12:81-88, 1971.
3. Yeng, M.C. and Hursch, C.: The use of a semi-Markov process for describing sleep patterns. Biometrics 29:667-676, 1973.
4. Cox, D.R.: Regression models and life-tables. J. R. Stat. Soc. 2:187-220, 1972.
5. Darwin, J.H.: Notes on a three-decision process for comparing two binomial populations. Biometrika 46:106-113, 1959.
6. Armitage, P.: Sequential Medical Trials. Oxford:Blackwell Scientific Publications, 1960.
7. Bross, I.: Sequential medical plans. Biometrics 8:188-205, 1952.
8. Elfring, G.L. and Schultz, J.R.: Group sequential designs for clinical trials. Biometrics 29:471-477, 1973.
9. Bray, D.F. and Lyon, D.A.: Three-class attributes plans in acceptance sampling. Technometrics 15:575-585, 1973.
10. Credeur, K.: Estimation from Incomplete Multinomial Data. Ph.D. thesis, Harvard University, Cambridge, Mass., 1978.
11. Kumbaraci, T.E.: The judgment of improvement — choice for decisions relating to medical efficacy. *In* Zeleny, M. (ed.): Multiple Criteria Decision Making. Columbia, S.C.:Univ. S.C. Press, 1972.
12. Kumbaraci, T.E.: Sequential evaluation of discretized parameters — an application to medical studies. Biometrics 29:842, 1973.
13. Kumbaraci, T.E.: Transitions in Trinomial data: A method for medical judgment. Biometrics 30:381, 1974.
14. Kumbaraci, T.E.: Tolerance limits over time — an exposition on acceptance. Trans. Am. Soc. Quality Control, 1976, p. 218.

A Microprocessor System To Measure Blood Pressure

D. H. Smith, J. S. Hutcheson, R. W. Lutz
and H. S. Hsiao

It is important to accurately measure blood pressure noninvasively both in clinical settings, such as routine monitoring of surgical patients in the operating and recovery rooms, and in experimental settings, such as monitoring of subjects during stress or exercise testing. This paper describes a system which measures blood pressure noninvasively. The system uses a microprocessor to control arm occlusion via cuff pressure and to detect Korotkoff (K) sounds only during a short window referenced to the EKG.

Background

There have been blood pressure systems described previously in the literature. Elder [1] reported on an all hardware, hard-wired system which operated in a single mode. A mode is defined here as the manner in which the cuff is inflated and deflated and the blood pressure reading is determined. To find systolic pressure, the cuff in Elder's system inflates to systolic pressure and tracks for 100 seconds. The cuff then deflates, gives the arm a rest and repeats the cycle. The system finds diastolic pressure in a similar manner.

Brener [2] also developed an all hardware, hard-wired system which operates in a dual cuff mode. One cuff records systolic pressure while the other cuff records diastolic pressure. The system uses automatic cuff inflation, K sound detection and mechanical pressure trip points.

D. H. Smith, J. S. Hutcheson, R. W. Lutz and H. S. Hsiao, The University of North Carolina, Chapel Hill.

Looney [3] described a microprocessor-based instrument which measures blood pressure from oscillations in cuff pressure. Operating in a single mode, this instrument looks for the lowest cuff pressure with the maximum oscillations. This pressure is output as the mean arterial pressure, and systolic and diastolic values are determined by extrapolation using the attenuation rate of the oscillations.

A disadvantage of all these previous systems is that each is limited to one or two modes of operation. For one to have the capability of choosing either to replicate the traditional auscultatory method used by physicians or to measure blood pressure more accurately or more rapidly, several modes are desirable. Another disadvantage of these systems is artifact susceptibility due to subject movement and surges in the pressure system. The system discussed here attempts to solve these problems by incorporating the following objectives: multiple modes of operation, improved artifact rejection and a fixed hardware design that will allow one to change from one mode to another, adjust control parameters, add a new mode or refine an existing mode via software. It also features portability and multiple outputs, including a front panel output for instant visual feedback, an analog output for chart recording and a digital output for communicating with digital peripheral devices.

System Hardware, Architecture and Operation

The system hardware components are described below:

1. The system is based on the KIM-1 microcomputer with its monitor in 2K of ROM (includes teletype and cassette tape routines) and with 1K of RAM. The system software is stored in a 2K EPROM on a peripheral circuit board. Both the keypad and the display are remoted to the front panel of the instrument and the display is divided into two groups of three digits for displaying systolic and diastolic pressures.

2. Two of the system's modes require two cuffs. Two sets of air valves — one set of three valves for each cuff — regulate inflation and deflation of the cuffs. Each set has an inflate/deflate valve, a fast/slow valve and a hold/release valve. By proper manipulation of these valves, either cuff can undergo

rapid inflation, slow inflation, rapid deflation or slow deflation; or, the pressure in the cuff can simply be maintained. The air valves are controlled through an optically isolated driver circuit. The optical isolation is to prevent malfunction of the system's integrated circuitry due to surges from the collapsing magnetic fields around the air valves.

3. Two model LX1702 G, 0-15 psi, National Semiconductor pressure transducers — one for each cuff — detect cuff pressure.

4. Another circuit board contains both the amplifier circuitry for the pressure transducers and the digital-analog conversion circuitry for the system's analog output.

5. A third circuit board serves as a data acquisition and memory board. The board contains two I/O ports, an eight channel multiplexer, an analog-digital converter, and a 2K EPROM in which the system software resides.

The block diagram in Figure 1 shows the system configuration. The system software is stored in the EPROM on the data acquisition card. The air valves are controlled through the KIM I/O port B. The pressure signals from the transducers are input to the system through the multiplexer, A/D converter and one of the I/O ports on the data acquisition card. The K sounds, detected and processed by a Parke-Davis portable electronic manometer, and the EKG are input through the other I/O port on the data acquisition card. The pressure reading is output to the KIM display and through the KIM port A to the D/A converters for analog recording.

The timing chart in Figure 2 illustrates the procedure used for artifact rejection. The first waveform shows a series of pulses which indicate the occurrence of the R wave of the EKG. As soon as an R wave is detected, a delay called K delay is initiated. The length of this delay is programmable. When K delay is over, K window begins. For a K sound to be detected, the leading edge of the K sound pulse must occur within this window. The length of the window is also programmable.

Figure 3 shows the flow chart for K sound detection. After the data are input, the routine interrogates the status of the K window. During the first pass through the K sound routine, the K window is not open; so, the routine checks for the occurrence of an R wave. If there is no R wave, registers are cleared and the

BLOOD PRESSURE MONITOR BLOCK DIAGRAM
KIM I
SYSTOLIC PRESS
DIASTOLIC PRESS
ADDRESS
CONTENT
I/O PORT A
8 BIT LATCH
K4 1ΦΦ1
8 BIT DIA CON-VER-TER
ANALOG SYSTOLIC PRESS
8 BIT LATCH
K4 1ΦΦ1
8 BIT DIA CON-VER-TER
ANALOG DIASTOLIC PRESS
TIMER CLOCK
I/O PORT B
NOT USER AVAIL-ABLE (CHIP SELECT)
INT
SOLENOID AIR VALVE DRIVER MODULE
AIR VALVE
AIR VALVE
AIR VALVE
TO SYSTOLIC CUFF
AIR VALVE
AIR VALVE
AIR VALVE
TO DIASTOLIC CUFF
ADDR BUS
DATA BUS
6530 K3
DATA ACQUISITION CARD
TIMER
I/O PORT
8 BIT A/D CON-VER-TER
8 CHAN MUX
EOC SC
SYSTOLIC PRESS
DIASTOLIC PRESS
LX1702A
LX1702A
0-255 mmHg
0-5 volts
NOT USED
E PROM 1KX8
K1
RAM 64X8
OA06
I/O PORT B
K SOUNDS SYSTOLIC
K SOUNDS DIASTOLIC
EKG

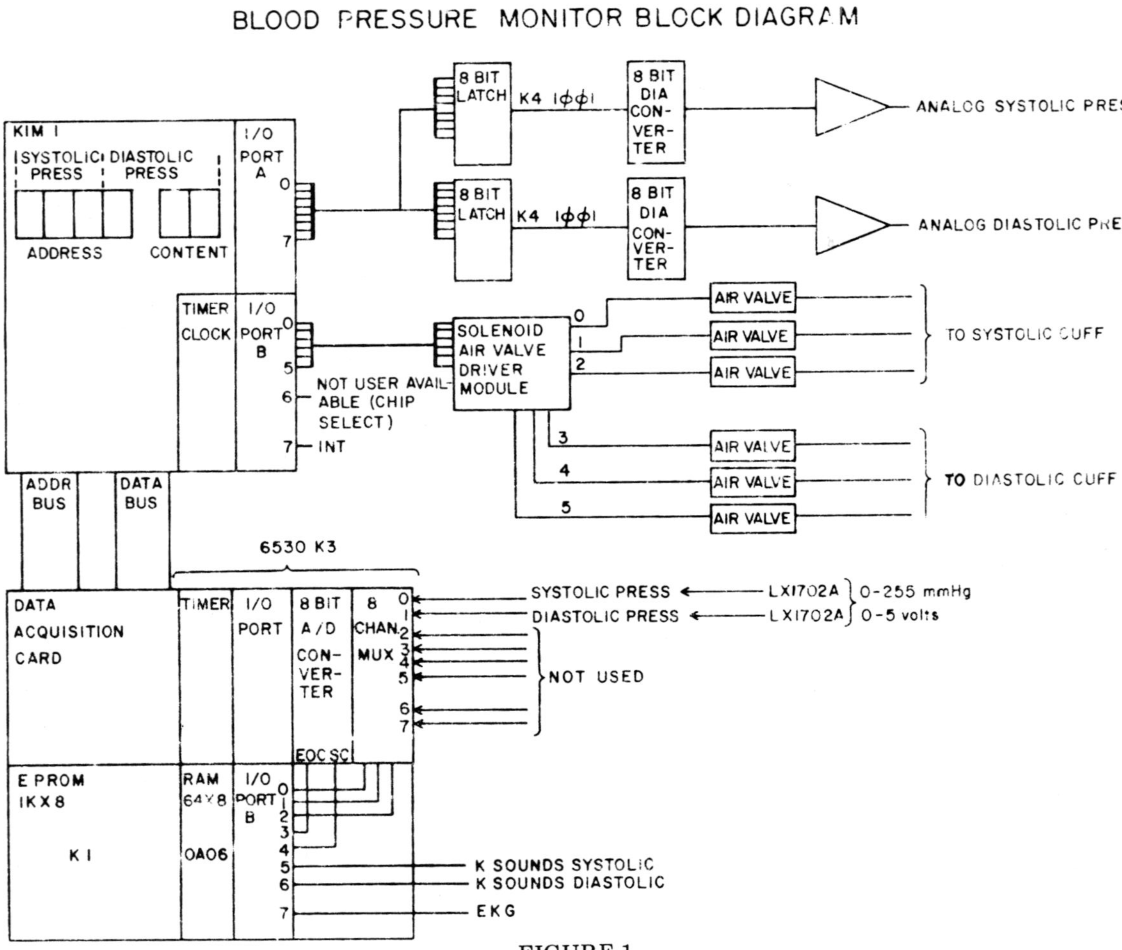

FIGURE 1.

TIMING CHART FOR K SOUND DETECTION
R WAVE
K DELAY
K WINDOW
K SOUND
R FLAG
K WINDOW FLAG
K FLAG

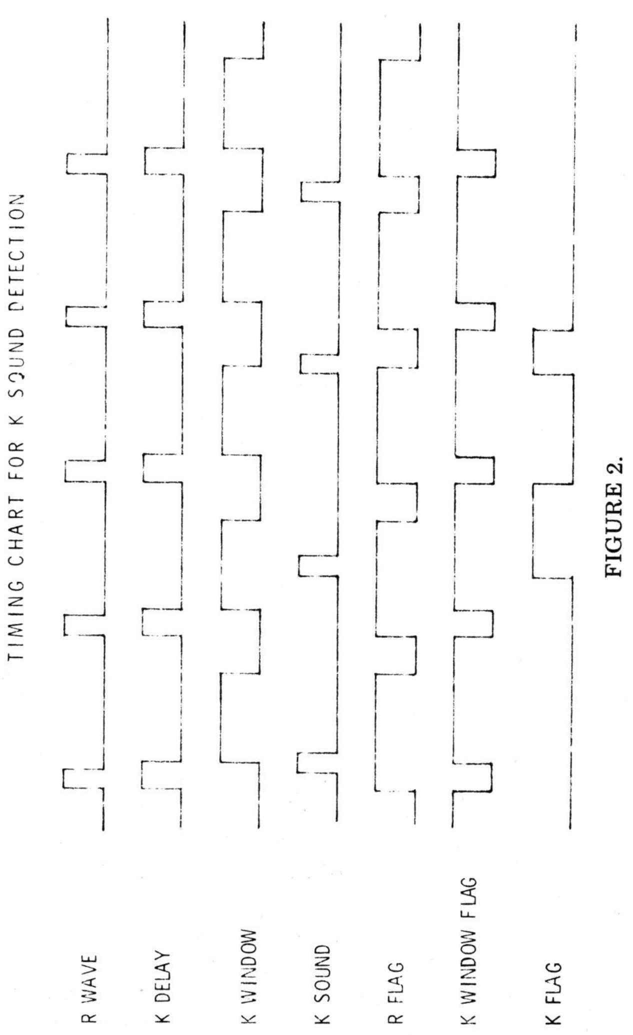

FIGURE 2.

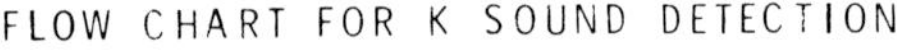

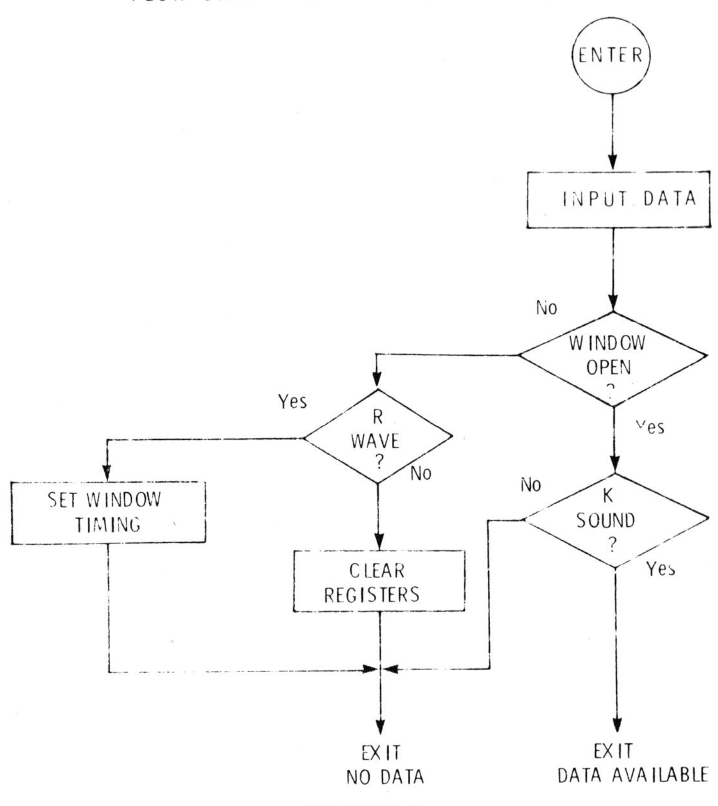

FIGURE 3.

routine is left with no data. If there is an R wave, the K window timing is initiated. During the next pass through the routine, the K window is open. If a K sound occurs, the routine records the pressure in the cuff. In this way, any artifact that occurs outside the window is rejected.

The system has multiple modes of operation:

1. Mode 1 is a single cuff mode in which the cuff is rapidly inflated to a programmable pressure greater than systolic pressure and then slowly deflated to a programmable pressure lower than diastolic pressure. During the slow deflate, the pressure in the cuff is recorded at every K sound occurrence. The first pressure recorded is taken as systolic pressure and the last one is taken as diastolic pressure. These pressure values are

displayed and there is a programmable delay after which the cycle is repeated. This mode corresponds to the traditional auscultatory method used by physicians.

2. Mode 2 is a single cuff mode in which the cuff is slowly inflated and pressure is displayed at the end of inflation; then, the cuff is slowly deflated and pressure is displayed at the end of deflation. There is a programmable delay and then the cycle repeats. This mode allows comparison of pressure values determined during inflation with those determined during deflation.

3. Mode 3 is a single cuff average mode which consists of slow inflate, slow deflate, average, display, delay and repeat. The pressure values recorded during inflation are averaged with those recorded during deflation. Pressure values read during an inflation only mode tend to be too high and those read during a deflation only mode tend to be too low. The purpose of this mode is that these differences will be averaged out to produce a slower, but more accurate blood pressure reading.

4. Mode 4 is a dual cuff tracking mode. One cuff inflates to near systolic pressure, tracks systolic pressure, deflates, displays, delays and then repeats. The other cuff similarly tracks diastolic pressure. This mode follows beat-to-beat changes in pressure over relatively short intervals.

5. Mode 5 is a dual cuff rapid sample mode. One cuff rapidly inflates above systolic pressure and then slowly deflates until the first K sound occurs. The system then rapidly deflates the cuff, displays the systolic pressure, delays and repeats the cycle. The other cuff rapidly inflates to just below diastolic pressure and then slowly inflates until the first K sound occurs. The system then rapidly deflates the cuff, displays the diastolic pressure, delays and repeats.

As a variation of mode 5, pulse transit time can be recorded and displayed along with either systolic or diastolic pressure. There is also a calibration mode which enables comparison of the system output with a known input pressure.

Tests and Results

Blood pressure readings have been obtained in the laboratory during body movements, running in place, tensing the arm and tapping on the cuff. The accuracy of this system's pressure readings is validated by comparing them with direct arterial pressure. Some preliminary data from one such pilot study are presented here.

Figure 4 shows some results of the single cuff average mode. The upper three lines are systolic pressure and the lower three are diastolic pressure. The solid line is direct arterial pressure. The dashed line represents the pressure values obtained by hand scoring the polygraph recording. The dash-dot line is the system display. The values recorded by the system were consistently below direct systolic pressure and above direct diastolic

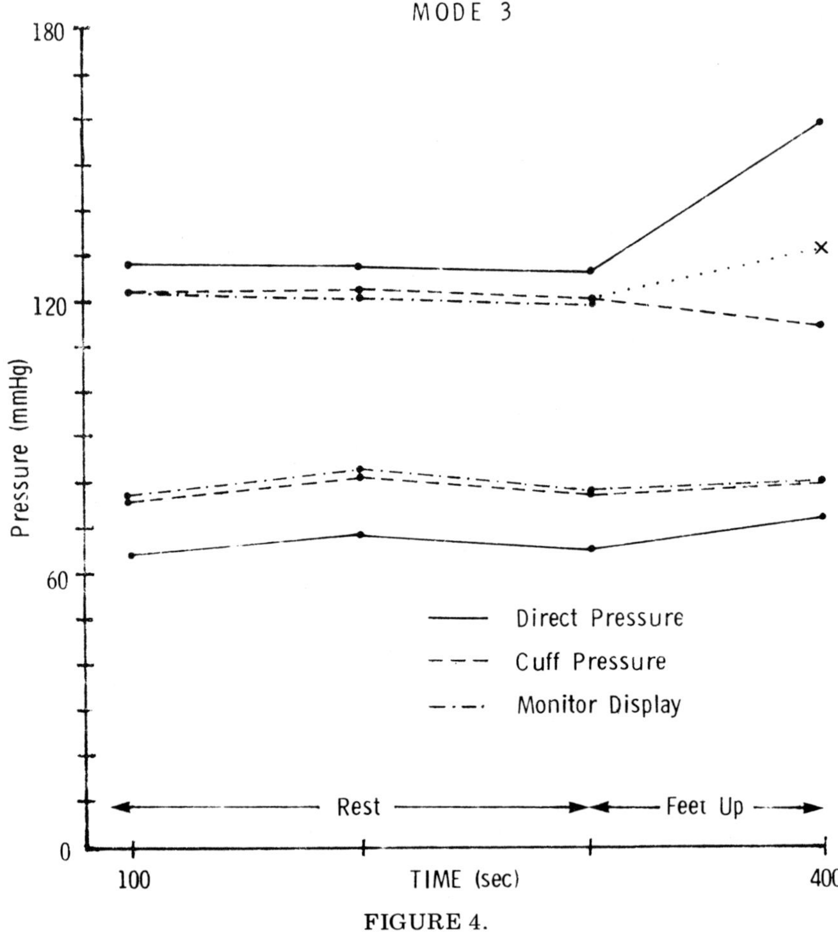

FIGURE 4.

pressure. This system's accuracy depends upon the ability of the Parke-Davis instrument to detect the K sounds. If the Parke-Davis instrument fails to detect the first K sound during deflation, this system will record a lower pressure than the actual pressure. The dotted line illustrates a point where the polygraph recording indicates that the Parke-Davis missed a K sound.

Figure 5 shows some data from the rapid inflate-slow deflate mode. Again, this system recorded values below direct

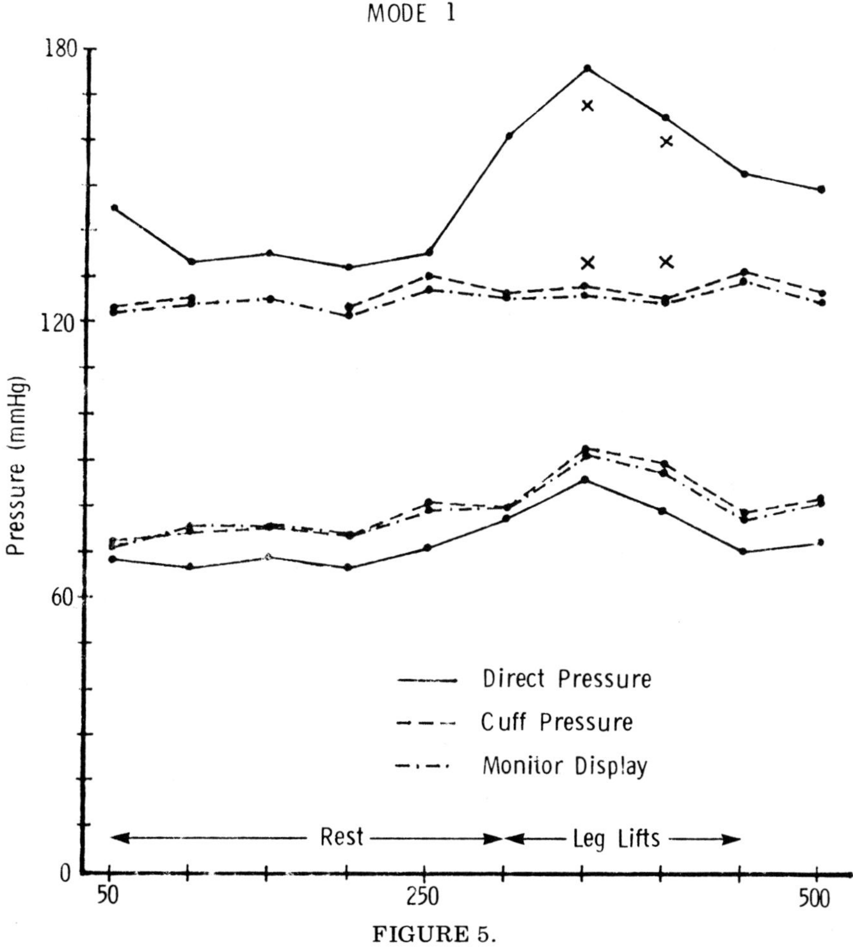

FIGURE 5.

systolic pressure and above direct diastolic pressure. The X's indicate suspect K sound detection.

Conclusion

In both these modes studied so far, the pressures from this system agree with the pressures from hand scoring. This system overcomes many of the disadvantages of other systems with its increased flexibility and relative insensitivity to movement artifact. However, there are some differences between the values obtained by this system and the direct pressures, which are at least partly due to the inability to reliably detect the K sounds at systole and diastole. A series of ten arterial punctures is planned to further validate the accuracy of the system and to compare the relative effectiveness of the various modes.

References

1. Elder, S.T., Longacre, A., Welsh, M.W. and McAfee, R.D.: Apparatus and procedure for training subjects to control their blood pressure. Psychophysiology, Vo. 14 No. 1, Jan. 1977.
2. Brener, J. and Kleinman, R.A.: Learned control of decreases in systolic blood pressure. Nature 226:1063-1064, 1970 (also, personal communication, 1972).
3. Looney, J.: Blood Pressure By Oscillometry. Medical Electronics, April 1978, p. 57.

Multiphasic Testing at Kaiser-Permanente

Morris F. Collen, M.D.

Introduction

In 1948, Breslow introduced "multiphasic" screening into a public health environment in San Jose, California. In 1951, the Kaiser-Permanente Medical Care Program initiated in San Francisco and Oakland the first multiphasic screening projects within a prepaid health plan (currently termed in the United States a Health Maintenance Organization).

However, when such a program has continuing responsibility for the medical care of a specific community or of a defined population, after the first screening for most chronic conditions (e.g., hypertension), further annual screening for undetected disease is often not cost-effective, since the majority of persons with chronic disease have been made aware of their condition on the first screen. Accordingly, the objective of periodic retesting is to provide continuing medical care for the chronic diseases and to monitor the status of the condition.

In 1963 to 1964, these original Oakland and San Francisco projects were replaced by the first automated "multiphasic health testing services" (MHTS) which have operated continuously since. These two MHTS programs currently examine more than 50,000 patients a year and since 1964 have provided more than 600,000 examinations.

These two programs have served as the base for extensive evaluation studies of MHTS. In summary, these evaluations have shown that it is the most cost-effective method of providing health examinations to a large population, it decreases costs of primary care by providing an alternative entry mode to a health

Morris F. Collen, M.D., Medical Methods Research, Oakland, Calif.

care system and it improves long-term outcome by decreasing mortality from potentially postponable conditions.

Based upon the demonstrated success of these MHTS models for preventive medical services in Oakland and San Francisco, other Kaiser-Permanente facilities now operate similar programs in Santa Clara, Redwood City, Sacramento, Walnut Creek, Los Angeles, San Diego, Portland, Cleveland and Honolulu.

Objectives of MHTS

MHTS within the Kaiser-Permanente program functions as an integral part of a health care delivery system and supports a variety of objectives:

1. Provide periodic health checkups for
   a. Health status evaluation (health appraisal).
   b. Health maintenance, monitoring and education (health promotion).
   c. Early disease detection for unknown conditions (case finding).
   d. Disease status monitoring for known conditions (disease monitoring).
2. Serve as an entry mode to the health care system (triage).
3. Serve as a referral laboratory for diagnostic surveys (diagnostic adjunct).
4. Provide hospital pre-admission examinations.
5. Improve quality of health care.
6. Decrease disability, morbidity and mortality.
7. Decrease costs of medical care.

Current Principles of Multiphasic Testing

There has developed a consensus that in accordance with the examinee's age, sex and specific risk factors, one should prescribe (a) a selective cost-effective set of tests and (b) a rational periodicity for re-examinations [1-4].

In Kaiser-Permanente, there are two processes available for providing the above: (a) traditional periodic health checkups and (b) periodic multiphasic health testing [5-12].

There is increasing support for taking a systems approach to personal preventive health care services. In contrast to the care of the sick, the care of the well is readily susceptible to a systems approach. Most people in a community are well; the "usual" person is not sick. Thus, "sick care" is for the exception to the usual. It is less suitable for programming and protocols and generally obtainable in good quality on an individual basis from physicians. Preventive health care or "well care" can be a routine, repetitive process, programmable for the usual person or even for everyone. Thereby, it is well suited for the application of protocols, automation and a systems approach, using allied health personnel trained in specific skills. This tends to exploit the economy of scale, the efficiency of automation and the quality assurance of control process monitoring; it can improve cost, service and quality.

A universal examination procedure for all people is, of course, not suitable. Which tests are cost-effective is dependent upon the sensitivity and specificity of the test, the cost of the test and the prevalence of the condition in the target population. Clearly, a system must be flexibly designed to select the most cost-effective test for each person. How often tests should be done depends upon the person's age and health status. Kaiser-Permanente has tested the value of urging annual check-ups, but has never advocated annual check-ups for all adults. Certainly the increasing incidence of disease with age indicates that older people need check-ups more frequently than those who are younger. Most "health monitoring" packages show considerable agreement on their recommendations. Kaiser-Permanente now generally advocates the following for screening of well persons: screening check-ups every three to five years for the 20s and 30s; every two to three years for the 40s; and every year or two after the 50s. For persons with clinically important abnormalities, disease monitoring check-ups should be obtained every year or as directed by their physician. Each Kaiser-Permanente MHTS has its own battery of tests tailored to the specific needs of its patient population and physician staff.

We have more than 25 years of experience with multiphasic health testing [5, 6]. Our experience shows that adults find such multiphasic check-ups to be very acceptable and that a substantial percentage voluntarily avail themselves of periodic health check-ups. Our studies have shown that this approach is very effective for early disease detection and health maintenance. For some asymptomatic conditions such as anemia, the great majority of patients and their physicians are unaware of the condition (78% "new"); whereas for most chronic conditions only about one fourth are newly detected and the majority return to MHTS for monitoring of the known disease. By appropriate selection of tests, which result in an acceptable cost per positive test (Table 1) [12], the process can be very cost-effective. Our studies have shown that such a systemized approach not only decreases the costs of the initial health status evaluation, but also decreases significantly the total costs of care (by about 20%) for at least one year, as compared to the traditional mode of the patient-physician encounter (Table 2) [7-9]. Urging periodic multiphasic check-ups decreases significantly the mortality for all over the age of 35 for some potentially postponable conditions to which the check-up is directed (Table 3); shows a lower mortality from all causes for those who elect to come in for check-ups as compared to those who do not (Table 4); and decreases disability and increases average net earnings for middle-aged men (Table 5) [5, 10, 11].

Table 1. Cost Per Positive Test by Age Group

	Under 40		*40-59*		*60 and Over*	
Test	*%+*	*$/+*	*%+*	*$/+*	*%+*	*$/+*
Blood pressure	0.4	88	4.3	8	11.5	3
EKG	10.2	9	17.7	5	31.5	3
Chest x-ray	2.1	69	7.4	20	19.2	8

Modified from Collen et al [12].

Table 2. Summary of 12-Month Total Resource Costs ($/Yr/1,000 Examinees, Adjusted for Age, Sex and Health Status)

	TMC	*MHT*
Physician costs (% of traditional)	93,673 (100)	68,714 (73)
Total costs (% of traditional)	131,179 (100)	105,966 (81)

Modified from Garfield et al [7].

Table 3. Deaths Per 1,000 Among 10,000 Kaiser-Permanente Members During 7 Years

	Check-ups Urged	*Check-ups Not Urged*
Potentially postponable	3.7	7.4
High blood pressure	.6	2.2
Bowel cancer	.4	1.8
All causes (including accidents)	35.6	39.2

Modified from Dales et al [10, 11].

Table 4. Mortality and Standard Mortality Ratios, All Subjects, 1965-1973

No. of MHTS 1965-1973	*Person-Years of Observation in This Category*	*Number of Deaths*	*Crude Mortality Deaths/1000 Person-Years*	*Standardized Mortality Ratio*
0	38384	310	8.08	1.38
1	19039	112	5.88	1.02
2	11189	51	4.56	0.74
3	7874	36	4.57	0.71
4-6	13282	59	4.44	0.62
7+	3959	13	3.28	0.40

Table 5. Cost-Benefit Analysis of Periodic MHT Examinations in Men (Ages 45-54 at Entry)

		1965	*1967*	*1969*	*1971*	*1965-1971 Total*
Percent of initial group with no disability	C	86.8	81.0	76.2	70.1	
	S	87.5	83.2	81.2	74.2	
Average annual earnings/man	C	$7038	$7350	$8271	$9270	
	S	$7083	$7488	$8510	$9371	
Average earnings net difference/man						$822

S = Study group of 1,229 men.
C = Control group of 1,364 men.
Modified from Collen [5].

Systemized health check-ups can effectively identify each person's health needs and arrange appropriate services to meet these needs. Selective testing applies acceptable criteria for test selection to identify high-risk persons and those who are early asymptomatic-sick. It then refers the sick to appropriate "sick care" services. The majority who are well can be referred to health education and health counseling services which try to further improve their current health status. This approach serves as an efficient entry mode to health care and provides each individual with the opportunity for assistance with categorical and lifestyle problems, such as stop-smoking programs.

Even though scientific efficacy of health check-ups has not been demonstrated to everyone's satisfaction, a significant percentage of Americans are already receiving medical check-ups, employment examinations and physical fitness appraisals, for one reason or another. Many are following the model set by our presidents, generals and industry executives for periodic health evaluations. It is not possible to isolate expenditures for well-person care in the course of physician office visits, but these expenses are already built into our nation's overall health care costs. Systemized health testing services, available to all people and all physicians in the community, would be much more efficient. At Kaiser-Permanente, these services and costs have been included since our inception; we believe this has been done in a very cost-effective manner and that this, in its own way, helps us compete successfully with alternative health care programs.

Since health status appraisals by a variety of modes are already built into our national health care costs and since there is more agreement than disagreement on which tests should be done and how often, we believe that a major issue is how our country should better organize its health care to provide check-ups. Our experience suggests that if governmental policy is to encourage and finance personal preventive health, it should support systemized approaches to personal preventive health services such as multiphasic health testing.

References

1. Task Force Reports. Preventive Medicine, USA. New York:PRODIST, 1976.

2. Conference on Health Promotion and Disease Prevention. Institute of Medicine, National Academy of Sciences, February 1978.
3. Nightingale, E.O. et al: Perspectives on health promotion and disease prevention in the U.S. A Staff Paper. Institute of Medicine, National Academy of Sciences, January 1978.
4. Breslow, L. and Somers, A.R.: A lifetime health-monitoring program. N. Engl. J. Med. 296:601-608, 1977.
5. Collen, M.F. (ed.): Multiphasic Health Testing Services. New York: John Wiley & Sons, 1978.
6. Collen, M.F.: A case study of multiphasic health testing. *In* Medical Technology and the Health Care System: A Study of Equipment-Embodied Technologies. The National Research Council's Committee on Technology and Health Care, National Academy of Sciences, 1978.
7. Garfield, S. et al: Evaluation of an ambulatory medical-care delivery system. N. Engl. J. Med. 294:426-431, 1976.
8. Collen, M.F.: Cost analyses of the Kaiser Foundation's systemized health evaluation. Preventive Medicine, USA. New York:PRODIST, 1976, pp. 706-714.
9. Collen, M.F. et al: Cost analyses of alternative health examination modes. Arch. Intern. Med. 137:73-79, 1977.
10. Dales, L.G., Friedman, G.D., Ramcharan, S. et al: Multiphasic checkup evaluation study: 3. Outpatient clinic utilization, hospitalization and mortality experience after seven years. Prev. Med. 2:221-235, 1973.
11. Dales, L.G., Friedman, G.D. and Collen, M.F.: Evaluation of a periodic multiphasic health checkup. Method. Inform. Med. 12:140-146, 1974.
12. Collen, M.F., Feldman, R., Siegelaub, A.B. and Crawford, D.: Dollar cost per positive test for automated multiphasic screening. N. Engl. J. Med. 283:459-463, 1970.

Multiphasic Health Screening at New York Telephone

G. H. Collings, Jr., M.D.

My own personal experience with Multiphasic Health Screening (MHS) encompasses a period of nearly 30 years. In the early years, we were concerned with the logistics, the mechanics and the methodology required to convert what up to that time had been monophasic screening programs (for example, tuberculosis detection) into multiple test systems. As for our expectation at that time in regard to what MHS would accomplish, we didn't give it much thought. In our experience with tuberculosis we had observed that if a case of this disease was detected, something would be done about it. From this, it was logical to assume that if a case of any other disease were detected, something would be done about it too. Furthermore, it was pretty much accepted as given that if a disease was found early in its course, there was a better chance for cure. It never occurred to us that individuals, when advised of positive findings, might procrastinate in taking corrective action or ignore the positive findings altogether. On the contrary, it was assumed that disease detection was tantamount to health improvement. Also, in the early days not much thought was given to the effectiveness of any particular test. If it measured something that was clinically significant, it was a candidate for inclusion. If a test could be done with a minimum of difficulty and if the out-of-pocket cost was reasonable, it was included.

As experience accumulated over the succeeding years, it became obvious that most of our assumptions were either totally false or at the very least required substantial modification. Moreover, by the end of the first decade we were well into

---

G. H. Collings, Jr., M.D., Corporate Medical Director, New York Telephone, New York, N.Y.

serious inquiry on the part of a number of investigators as to the appropriateness of some of the widely used tests, and the first of studies to quantify the complex relationships between specific tests and the diseases they identified had begun to emerge.

By the mid 1960s, MHS had become widely discussed and numerous MHS programs had been begun or were about to begin. Those in the business of selling automated systems or wishing to get into that business were eyeing MHS as a potentially lucrative market for all kinds of technical gear and/or complete screening systems. At that time those with experience with MHS could have told you that successful use of MHS for health improvement depended upon two factors: (1) efficient identification of disease with emphasis on the word "efficient" and (2) effective follow-up and correction of the disease found. However, many of the MHS programs around the country at that time failed to recognize the importance and interdependence of these two objectives, and most ignored the second one completely. This was a fatal mistake which was to result in the failure of many MHS efforts and encouraged a wave of critical and, I believe, unwarranted commentaries on the fundamental lack of validity of the MHS concept itself.

When we began to construct the New York Telephone MHS program about 10 years ago, we had the advantage of 15 years of experience with the evolution of MHS in other contexts and were well aware of the twin requirements for efficient detection and effective follow-up. Consequently, special attention was given to designing a system that would encourage continuing efficiency and improvement in disease detection and, more importantly, would emphasize follow-up to achieve real disease correction and health improvement as the primary priority.

During the succeeding ten years we have learned what can and cannot be expected from MHS when properly conceived, implemented and managed as applied to a stable industrial population.

There has been a steady (about 10% year over year) improvement in the efficiency with which we can run the MHS system. This gain has come more from learning how to better manage the system than from any major technological breakthroughs in test methods or clinical capabilities. Improved test application, more sophisticated standard setting, more effective educational and promotional methods, a thorough understanding of the interplay between true positives and false positives and true and false negative test results (the so-called test sensitivity vs. test specificity), more selective identification of populations or subpopulations to be screened, more advanced automation of both the information gathering and the information processing procedures and other aspects of improved system management have combined to permit earlier, more accurate and less costly detection of disease. The cost has progressively decreased over the years.

We have also been quite successful with respect to follow-up and correction of detected disease. Probably the best measure of success in this regard is the percent of conditions corrected but before I pursue that further, let me mention a number of natural factors which singly or in combination tend to prevent successful disease correction in the contemporary world of patient and physician behavior.

First, the physician resents the intrusion of a third party-multiphasic health screener into what he considers his private domain. Second, even after the physician is persuaded to accept the possibility that his patient may have a previously unrecognized abnormality, the first thing that he does is to repeat all the positive tests in a different laboratory. When the repeat tests do not confirm the abnormality, the credibility of the MHS program is impugned and its further effectiveness in working toward health improvement for that individual is minimized. Third, private physicians who deal daily with severe disease are likely not to be impressed by test abnormalities in the borderline or moderately elevated ranges and are likely to advise against any further attention in these cases, thus effectively blocking any corrective action. Finally, the patient is likely to procrastinate both in going to the physician in the first place and in following his advice when it is given. Getting patients to follow even a simple routine of pill taking over a long period of time is recognized as difficult to accomplish, and getting the patient to modify established life style is even more difficult. These and other similar factors tend to defeat attempts to get effective action taken for positive findings from MHS. As a matter of fact, experience has shown that without significant effort to offset these natural factors not much in the way of health improvement happens. MHS disease detection, standing alone, with no attention to follow-up beyond notification of the patient and/or his physician will under ordinary circumstances not achieve correction of more than 10% to 15% of correctable conditions.

It was just this situation that the New York Telephone MHS program was designed to remedy. Over a period of years by diligent and persistent attack on this problem we have been able to substantially improve the results achieved. The initial year or two of operation resulted in the improved yield to 30% to 35% correction of correctable conditions. However, over the subsequent seven or eight years, we were able to further raise these figures to about 50% by improved management of the system. Impressive as these gains are, toward the end of this period it became obvious that as long as the MHS program was coupled to the existing community medical care system and dependent upon it for corrective action, it was unlikely that any further improvement could be achieved. In other words correction of about 50% of correctable conditions was nearly maximum.

Moreover, by this time another important understanding was emerging from our experience. Those MHS tests and procedures most effective in obtaining the eradication of *existing* disease were usually the least effective in the prevention of *future* disease or the improvement of current *health*. Consequently, the better we managed in the interest of improving the former, the worse things got vis-a-vis the latter. This incongruity, plus a number of other considerations too complex to discuss here, eventually led to the emergence of the concept of Health Care Management (HCM) as a more attractive alternative to MHS for the purpose of health improvement in an industrial population.

We are now embarked upon an extensive effort to work out the detailed methods for HCM and to apply this new technique to our objective of health improvement. The fact that more advanced systems are evolving for industry's specific purposes should not be interpreted, however, as categorical indictment of MHS in industry. On the contrary, we have shown to our own satisfaction that MHS when run properly can contribute substantially to disease detection and correction and that it is satisfactorily cost-effective even though full correction of all correctable conditions is not achieved.

The First Ten Years of The Society for Advanced Medical Systems

(Establishmentarianism Recapitulates Ontogeny)

Dean F. Davies, M.D.

Ontogeny is the "origin and development of the individual organism." The establishment of the Society for Advanced Medical Systems has recapitulated this familiar process. Thus, SAMS had parents, it was conceived, went through gestation, was born, had an infancy and grew through virility to maturity. It had flirtations with other organizations and, like people, has sometimes had identity problems.

Every historian necessarily puts his own stamp on the history he writes no matter how objective he tries to be. And so it will be with the historical account of SAMS. Clearly, many things happened during the past ten years which had great impact on the history of the organization; no individual was present or informed about all of them. However, it is appropriate that I tell the story of its early days from first-hand knowledge and supplement the remainder of the story from the memory and records of others.

Organizationally, SAMS was the foster-child of the Engineering Foundation Conferences on Biology and Medicine. In July 1967 the Foundation had held a four day meeting in multiphasic health testing in Milwaukee, Wisconsin. Some of the early members of SAMS attended that meeting, but SAMS had not yet been conceived. In fact, there was hardly a "boy meets girl" relationship since the physicians could not be distinguished from the engineers at that meeting.

Dean F. Davies, M.D., Life Extension Institute, New York, N.Y.

I had not heard of that meeting although I had been interested enough in multiphasic health testing to have spent ten days studying Morris Collen's facility at Kaiser-Permanente and was slated to head up a screening unit for Columbia University at Harlem Hospital. By the fall of 1967 I had been offered and accepted a Professorship of Preventive Medicine at the University of Tennessee in Memphis. In putting together an application to the Memphis Regional Medical Program for a demonstration grant I discovered that the Engineering Foundation was planning a second meeting on multiphasic health testing to be held at Procter Academy, Andover, New Hampshire, during the week of August 5, 1968. Since I had not received an invitation I assumed it was for an exclusive "in" group but I managed to obtain an invitation anyway. The theme of the meeting was "Physical Parameters in Multiphasic Screening."

Within hours of my arrival at Procter Academy two things impressed me. First, name tags did not indicate degrees, profession or institution so I did not know whether I was, except for Cesar Caceres, the only physician or whether there were others. The second impression was best expressed in a letter I later wrote to Robert Westlake, a past-president of the American Society of Internal Medicine and a speaker at the Andover meeting. In it I said: "At the risk of oversimplifying, it seems that industries, such as aerospace etc., are ready to devise and mass produce a system of multiphasic health screening." I recall that my gut feeling was the conviction that the effort of the engineers would be wasted unless the medical profession was involved at the outset. I was sure that the human, rather than the technological problem was not being reckoned with.

As for my first impression, in order to satisfy my curiosity about physicians in attendance I wondered out loud to a few strangers how many physicians they thought were in attendance. One was Marshall Driggs, M.D., and the other was Larry Taylor, an osteopathic physician from California. A third who joined us was Robert Katase, M.D. The thought that the engineers didn't know how important physician acceptance would be struck a responsive chord among the others and we went into a caucus. We determined to ask all interested physicians to come to a meeting to explore the need for an organization which would bridge the gap between medicine and technological sciences. It was suggested that Cesar Caceres, the Chairman of the Conference, be asked to make the announcement. He did and 29 of some 35 physicians attended the first of two meetings for the purpose. The second meeting held on August 8 was attended by 13. An organizing committee was elected consisting of Drs. Caceres, Driggs, Katase, Kirkham and Kopp with Davies as Chairman. This organizing committee was authorized to:

1. Gather information and report on what other physician groups were doing.
2. Proceed as indicated by these results.
3. Organize a meeting for the group at the American Public Health Association Convention in Detroit in November.

Naming the Little Tyke

You recall that the Andover meeting ended August 9, 1968. It is significant in the history of SAMS that as early as August 16 I wrote the members of the organizing committee, suggesting that the name of the new organization be "Medical Liaison Council on Health Protection Systems." By September 11 I was writing Marshall Driggs as follows:

> "The name has not been finalized; although the majority have approved Medical Liaison Council on Health Protection Systems, one thinks it is too long. I believe that Society for Health Protection Systems should be acceptable to all."

Marshall concurred. By October 4 I was writing Morris Collen that "the latest thinking is that a Society for Health Protection Systems or Advanced Medical Systems with medical leadership is needed." The final choice made at Detroit on November 14 was at least in part due to the fact that the acronym SAMS would make a good nickname.

There was never any doubt that the organization should be broader than multiphasic health testing and should bridge a communication gap between the engineering and the medical disciplines. The real problem was the need to make the medical community aware of what experts in technology could do.

By November 14 we had held the meeting at the Sheraton Cadillac in Detroit with 21 persons attending or represented.

Cesar Caceres was made pro-tem President. Other officers were Davies, President-elect; Vice-president for Automated Multitest Systems — Morris Collen; for Computer Technology — G. Octo Barnett; Laboratory Automation — Bill Kirkham; and for Advisory Boards and Councils — Gil Collings; Secretary — Bob Katase; and Treasurer — Marshall Driggs. Eighteen additional persons were elected to the Board.

It is of particular interest that "manpower development and integration of technology and allied health personnel" were incorporated as objectives of the Society at this first organizing meeting.

The fledgling Society was already invited to co-sponsor with the Engineering Foundation Research Conference a meeting called "Multiphasic Screening III" to be held in Deerfield, Massachusetts in August 1969. A meeting of the Executive Committee was held three weeks later at the Union League Club in New York. It was attended by Drs. Caceres, Davies, Driggs, Day, Kirkham, Greberman, Miller, Collings and Katase. Drs. Kirkham and Collings were appointed to a Constitution and By-laws Committee. Davies, Katase and Greberman made up the Nominating Committee. The President was authorized to appoint six additional standing committees and ad hoc committees as necessary.

Whether the brain-child, SAMS, was conceived in or out of the wedlock of Roberts Rules of Order is a moot question, but there is no question that conception took place in an intellectually orgiastic peak experience. There is also no question that the pregnancy was short; perhaps SAMS was a preemie. And the labor pains, unlike ontogeny, were distributed among a large number of enthusiastic parents.

First Annual Meeting

The August 1969 meeting, being sponsored jointly with the Engineering Foundation, was designated the first annual meeting of the Society. It covered national and international developments in screening; structure of engineering and medical societies; cost and benefit of screening; acceptance of screening by clients and by physicians' groups; and several other practical concerns with screening.

Things slowed for a while after the successful Deerfield meeting. Before discussing the subsequent Annual Meetings I would like to comment on how SAMS was brought up. You might consider the Deerfield meeting to be the birth cries of a healthy, bouncing — and legitimate — baby, because the knot had been tied; incorporation papers had been signed in May 1969. Kirkham worked it out in Pound Ridge, New York with attorney Alexander Bills. Kirkham and Collings had hammered out an excellent set of bylaws by January 11, 1969.

How long would it take the child to stand alone and take its first faltering steps? On September 30, 1970, with considerable help from Dr. Richard Hsieh, Chief of the Health Services Research and his staff at Baltimore's U.S. Public Health Service Hospital, SAMS first stood alone with a scientific program of ten papers and a business meeting. The Proceedings were later published and distributed to those who attended the meeting. There had been no general invitation to attend and the audience was largely composed of U.S.P.H.S. Hospital employees and Board members.

Coming of Age

If the organization SAMS is considered to be the organism, then it needed all the nurturing it could get from its family. So much attention was focused on the baby that adequate recognition was never given to many persons who fed and clothed it. To name any would be to slight others, but the first steps were taken only because of the tremendous effort and support of many persons. Because of this effort, SAMS was not just walking but was off and running at the third annual scientific meeting at the Albert Pick Hotel in Memphis. I sent notices to some 1,500 persons and the response was disturbingly gratifying because Marshall Driggs, as President-elect and Program Chairman, had not finalized the program. As a medical diplomat he had persuaded Wesley Hall, President of the American Medical Association, to talk at the Plenary Session. Lester Goodman, Sidney Garfield, Anne Somers, Morris Collen and Bob Westlake were added to the Plenary Sessions. Attendance was just under 100 and the enthusiasm was contagious; they liked the colloquia in which specific issues were addressed.

In this "damn the torpedoes" atmosphere — and in my innocence — I made a promise that the proceedings of the meeting would be published. The Board had not authorized it and at that time couldn't afford it, but a promise was a promise and I paid it. Without the proceedings the meeting came out well in the black. The highlight for me personally was the warm response my Presidential Address received. The day and a half follow-up Institute on Medical Information Systems for Medical Centers and Private Practice which the RMP and the University of Tennessee's Division of Continuing Education co-sponsored was also a success.

From the very beginning the Board had visions of a large organization with over 500 members and fellows, a newsletter and a journal and regional meetings during the year. Our first announcement was a brochure printed while Cesar Caceres was President. It listed the aims of the Society and on the next page said:

> "INNOVATIVE COMMUNICATIONS. This inclusive concept permits SAMS to evolve a dynamic program consisting of Monthly Bulletin . . .Monograph Series; Information and Advisory Service; Tapes, Audiovisuals, Programmed Learning; Continuing Education Programs; Interdisciplinary Dialogue; Handbooks and Directories."

It also contained the names of the officers, Board and Committee members and a mailing slip for those interested in more information. We were anxious to start a journal and a newsletter and easily found persons anxious to provide them at prices we couldn't afford. At one point I busied myself with doodling up a complex logo which the Board proceeded wisely to reject.

If we were overly ambitious and more imaginative than fiscally responsible at times, we believed that if there were nothing ventured there would be nothing gained. (I know at least one organization that has existed for over four years. It is not in debt but it has never had even a Board meeting!)

Memberships and applications for Fellowships started coming in after the Announcement and brochure were mailed out. A careful system of review of the credentials of fellowship applicants was followed. Checks for dues began arriving during 1969, 1970 and continued in 1971. In the absence of a secretariat it was almost predictable that problems would arise because of changing officers dispersed over the country, each volunteering all the time he could squeeze out of an already loaded schedule.

It is to Marshall Driggs' everlasting credit that he obtained the part-time services of SAMS' den mother, Pat Horner, at AIBS. According to Kirkham's treasurer's report there was $636 on hand in July 1970. By October 1971 we had received $4,087 in dues and went into the meeting in October with $2,260.

If SAMS showed his virility in Memphis, he demonstrated his maturity during each subsequent year, even the year he caught the "Money flu" (flew). But that is another story.

In October Driggs became President and Charles Weller, Conference Chairman. At this point some of my information becomes second-hand. To do justice to all Presidents I have solicited their assistance to provide highlights of their experience with SAMS. Pat Horner also was helpful in providing a structure of major events.

During 1972 SAMS was big enough to carry its weight in co-sponsoring the Health Delivery Year 2000 with the Engineering Foundation. Horner Associates became the secretariat. The Life Paid-up Membership was established so that SAMS could receive a transfusion (or infusion) of extra cash when it most needed it. The Fourth Annual Meeting at the Marriott in Rutherford had Larry Weed as its keynote speaker and again had the President of the American Medical Association.

SAMS again moved to a higher plateau when Morris Collen gave it the stature of an equal participant with ORSA (Operations Research Society of America) and Salutis Unitas (translated as Unity for Health), an international organization with headquarters near Rome, Italy. The Kaiser Foundation contributed heavily and loaned its beautiful facilities for this International Conference, SAMS' Fifth Annual Meeting.

The following year, 1974, was our sixth annual meeting and it again went to the home territory of the President. Charles Flagle had the distinction of being the first nonphysician President. Following Morris Collen's lead he chaired the Conference Committee as well. The theme was "Advanced Medical Systems: Issues and Challenges" and the successful meeting led to an end of the fiscal year well in the black.

In 1975 the pattern was broken momentarily. The meeting site was not on the home turf of the President, Charles Weller, and the Conference Chairman was neither President nor President-elect. I don't know whether this had anything to do with the fact that the notices of the meeting arrived late and the program, when it arrived, had fascinating titles but no names of presenters of papers. This was the first meeting I did not attend but from the record I gather that the fiscal year ended with a deficit. This was the year that the "money flew" virus got SAMS.

Something needed to be done. The Board bit the bullet and assessed each Board member $200. The President, Gilbeart Collings, finalized an affiliation with the Journal of Medical Systems and accomplished a number of other innovations. Edward Hinman as President-elect chaired the Conference Committee. As a full member of the Annual Conference on Engineering in Medicine and Biology SAMS was scheduled to meet in conjunction with the ACEMB in Boston. Our Eighth Annual Conference was co-sponsored with the Sixth Annual Conference of the Society for Computer Medicine. This put us back in the black.

Having joined the family of organizations belonging to the Annual Conference on Engineering in Biology and Medicine, SAMS joined the family reunion again in November 1977 in Los Angeles. The theme was Prospects and Challenges and Hinman, as President, gave the keynote address. As a result of efforts of Board Member Steve Metropoulos, Hinman and a prodigious amount of work by Pat Horner and her staff an application to the Department of Labor's Bureau of Apprenticeship and Training for a project for "Allied Health Apprenticeship and Training — A New Initiative" was approved and a contract awarded to SAMS by the government. This was not an inheritance but a special job. Executive Director Pat Horner, as Project Director of the contract, was delighted that SAMS had shown himself deserving of this responsibility.

SAMS has never been wealthy but it has not been fat with an excess of members either. At one time in 1970 a budget was prepared estimating an annual expense of $30,000 for which either 600 members (Fellows) at $50 each or 3,000 members at $10 would be required. Since 1971 there have been between

100 and 150 Fellows and we have had from 200 to 280 members. These have fluctuated, but we cannot really measure SAMS by height, weight and pocketbook. I do want to discuss his character.

First, I am unabashed in saying that I have never failed to come away from a Board meeting without a feeling of inspiration and admiration for the wisdom manifest in the corporate mind of its members. The whole is greater than the sum of its parts because the parts, the persons who have steered the Society, have themselves been highly intelligent, highly motivated and expert in a systems approach to issues. It is rare for me to stand in awe of persons or groups, but I continue to be impressed with the constant climb to higher plateaus that SAMS has backpacked.

One more word. I have been demonstrating by repeated analogies that the establishmentarianism of creating the Society for Advanced Medical Systems (SAMS) recapitulates the ontogeny of human development. There is a place that the analogy breaks down. SAMS does have a history of conception, birth, childhood, youth and maturity. But mere humans are mortal. SAMS has indefinite viability. You and I, through SAMS, in any contribution we have made will be surviving.